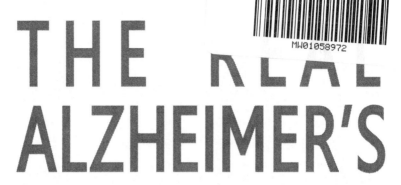

THE REAL ALZHEIMER'S

A Guide for Caregivers That Tells It Like It Is

With best wishes,
Suzanne Giesemann

Suzanne Giesemann

One Mind

www.OneMindBooks.com

Interior design by Linda Morehouse, webuildbooks.com
Cover design by Elisabeth Giesemann
Individuals depicted in the images are models and used for illustrative purposes only.

Library of Congress Control Number: 2012912453

Library of Congress Cataloging-in-Publication Data
The Real Alzheimer's: A Guide for Caregivers That Tells it Like it Is/Suzanne Giesemann

ISBN: 978-0-9838539-2-3

Printed in the United States of America

Published by One Mind Books: www.OneMindBooks.com

For the caregivers.
May you feel the love that surrounds you always
and know that you do not walk this path alone.

Acknowledgments

What makes *The Real Alzheimer's* special is the honesty of each story. The people on these pages are so very *human*. In one sense, they are strangers to us, but in another sense, they could be our next door neighbors. Many of them are, in fact, my neighbors. These beautiful souls invited me into their homes and into the most intimate corners of their lives for one simple reason: to help others who are on the same journey find their way more easily.

The professional caregivers featured here chose their vocation. They, like all those who make it their life's work to serve, deserve our utmost gratitude. The unpaid caregivers featured here did not choose this path, nor did their loved ones afflicted with dementia. They could have retreated into the solitude of what can be a very isolating disease. Instead, they stepped forward, opening their hearts to lessen the burden of those who walk the same path. I thank all of you for your courage and your trust. In sharing so honestly, you have made a difference.

At the risk of singling out any of the contributors, I especially thank Judy Simms. She is not a fictitious person, but one very real *character* with more guts, hutzpah, and compassion than I have ever encountered bundled into one spunky woman. She will stand up for what's right and she will stand and hold the hand of anyone in need. Judy, I stand and I salute you. Without you, this book would not have been written.

CONTENTS

* Names have been changed

FOREWORD

"ALZHEIMER'S SUCKS."

My patient, Ken, had early-onset Alzheimer's disease and made this proclamation at one of his appointments. He could no longer shave or dress himself, but somehow this was still clear in his deteriorating brain. As a memory disorders specialist at the University of South Florida, I took care of Ken from the time he was an avid cyclist with mild forgetfulness until his final, unconscious days in hospice and could not agree with him more.

The real Alzheimer's indeed "sucks." It robs us of our memories, steals our loved ones from us, and feeds into depression, stress, and family discord. When Suzanne Giesemann asked me to write a foreword for her book on the subject, I jumped at the chance. It would give me a chance to champion the voices of the true "experts" in the disease—the people who live with it every day.

The Real Alzheimer's is an emotional journey through this devastating disease through the eyes of caregivers, patients, and professionals. Every person's story is different, yet they all share common themes of loss, guilt, and sadness, as well as love, hope, and friendship. In my career, I have heard hundreds of stories like the ones in this book. Yet with each one, I come away with some small piece of information that can be useful to pass on to someone else. If you are reading this as a caregiver or family member of an Alzheimer's patient, heed the warnings to seek early treatment, take care of legal paperwork as soon as possible, and find a support group. If you have a friend or neighbor who is dealing with caregiving duties, offer specific assistance (like "Why don't I come over on Thursday mornings so you can go out?") and try to overlook behaviors that may be out of the ordinary. Many people find that their circle of friends dwindles when Alzheimer's appears; this just adds to stress. Rather than running away, try being patient, non-judgmental, and supportive. Never forget that there is still a person in there, as you'll read in chapter 17. Through the narratives shared in *The Real Alzheimer's*, you will gain insight into what it is like to wake up to this illness on a daily basis, and learn from others' mistakes and successes.

I keep a picture of Ken on my desk. It is the photo from the back of the booklet at his memorial service. In it, he is smiling brightly, walking his beloved dog. *Still a person.* I keep it there to motivate me—to work harder to intervene early, to practice empathy and patience, to tirelessly test new drugs in search of a cure. But I also keep it there because to me, his is the face of the real Alzheimer's. His. Nancy's. Tom's. Adele's. Desmond's. In this book, the names may be different, but the experiences are not unique. Suzanne Giesemann has done a wonderful job collecting the stories of real people and their very real experiences. This is The Real Alzheimer's.

Amanda G. Smith, MD
Medical Director
USF Health Byrd Alzheimer's Institute
Tampa, Florida

PREFACE

A KIDNAPPING. That's what it felt like.

I had known my neighbors Ava and Andrew for three years. In that time I watched Andrew's abilities steadily decline as Alzheimer's disease transformed him from a capable adult to a dependent child. Over the course of our acquaintance, I never saw his wife of ten years treat him with anything but tenderness and loving concern. I would see them walk hand-in-hand to the post office or sit side-by-side in a restaurant as Ava tried to bring as much normalcy as possible into their lives.

On this particular day it was Ava who needed care and concern as her life—already unsettled by her husband's disease—unraveled even more. I stood at her side as two men silently carried Andrew's belongings out the door. Andrew had been whisked away an hour earlier with the first load of boxes to avoid his confused questioning.

The taller of the two men was a hired hand. He seemed to have figured out that he'd gotten himself into something uncomfortable. He kept his eyes lowered as he traipsed in and out of the house. The second perpetrator was Andrew's son, a grown man who had taken his father to an attorney during a surprise visit from out of town several years earlier. Without saying a word to his step-mother, he had convinced Andrew to sign a durable power of attorney giving all responsibility for his care and his money to himself.

When the lawyer's letter arrived advising Ava that Andrew's son would be permanently taking her husband to live with him in his home, it was eleven days before Christmas. If Ava had any thought of fighting the legality of a document signed by a man who had been officially diagnosed with Alzheimer's disease, she would have to wait until after the holidays. In the meantime, she had seven days' notice to say goodbye to her husband, ho ho ho.

Bewildered and beaten down after being the full-time care-giver to a man who could no longer find his way to the bathroom or dress himself, Ava had asked me to be with her that day for moral support. She also invited Judy Simms, the facilitator of an Alzheimer's support group that Ava had been attending for some time. The three of us said nothing to the two men as they carried armfuls of Andrew's books, clothes, and furnishings past us. Once out of earshot, however, Judy launched a full-barrel assault at me.

"You have to write a book about this," she said, her eyes flash-ing behind a pair of small school-marm glasses. "This is just one story of thousands I could tell you."

As an author, people often suggested new book topics to me. I had several projects already in the works, and I had no intention of starting another. "Aren't there plenty of books out there already?" I asked Judy.

She shook her head.

"There's not enough education about what it's really like to help someone with Alzheimer's. We need a book to educate the caregivers and other people dealing with this disease. They just don't understand. The books that are out there are full of good in-formation," Judy said, "but many find them too clinical . . . too struc-tured. If you're in a crisis situation, you're too busy getting through the day to read a textbook."

I sighed, but Judy must have sensed that I was wavering. She reloaded and came at me from a different angle.

"Did you know that every 70 seconds someone in this country is diagnosed with Alzheimer's? By 2050 it's going to be every 33 seconds."

She paused a moment to let that sink in, then said, "And did you know that seventy percent of caregivers die before the one who has Alzheimer's?"

"How is that possible?" I asked, but the question seemed rhe-torical as my eyes fell on Ava's deeply drawn face.

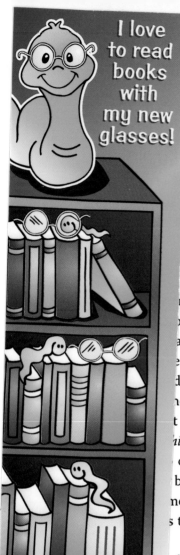

I love to read books with my new glasses!

said, confirming my suspicions. "These

with that one, hitting me square in the

in the gaps between Andrew's son and

e and Ava regaled me with stories. I

her husband, Chuck, to Alzheimer's.

st Ava's support group, but another at

ares her lessons-learned-the-hard-way

the long journey.

Judy said. "You read the checklists in

, and you think you're prepared, but you

ing to do. Never."

and like a stop sign. "When you find out

eimer's, they tell you to expect *this*, and

d her right index finger to the tip of each

e talked.

t like that. It's completely unpredictable.

is, and *this*." She spread her fingers wide

depressions she'd created. "Most of us

by day. It's not like you read in the books.

ner's."

s the words fell from her lips. "That's the

ed.

e book—*The Real Alzheimer's*."

"So you're going to write it?" Ava asked.

Judy clapped her hands like a kid, and I nodded my head in surrender.

It didn't take long to learn why Judy was so passionate about her work. One week later I sat with her in a support group meeting and felt the distress of the caregivers. I also felt the love and compassion they had for each other.

Most of those present were eager to talk with me. They wanted to do anything they could to help others dealing with the problems they faced every day. One woman, however, looked at me through narrowed eyes.

"I don't mean to insult you," she said with undisguised disdain, "but you can't write a book like this. The books you've written are all about things you know. You don't know anything about this."

By then I had already considered that problem. There were plenty of professionals with far more expertise and experience in the field of Alzheimer's than I who could write this book. My area of expertise was writing from the heart. Well aware of the stress the woman was under, I smiled at her with as much love as I could muster and explained, "I'm not going to tell what it's like to live with Alzheimer's. All of *you* are. This book is going to be told in the words of those who are dealing with it every day. That's the *real* Alzheimer's."

And that's what you'll find on the pages that follow. This book is not the result of in-depth research, nor does it contain summaries of the latest studies. It doesn't relate one person's isolated story, but shares, instead, a series of chats with those who are on the front lines—from the caregivers to the practitioners, and the patients themselves. Here you'll find a cross section of the population, because Alzheimer's isn't selective. Like a destructive storm, it affects a wide swath of society indiscriminately—high income and low, well-educated and street-smart.

You'll hear from husbands, wives, sons, daughters, and others caring for loved ones in the mild, moderate, and late stages of Alzheimer's. You'll read the rest of Ava and Andrew's story, of course, but you'll also hear from over a dozen others who are fighting their own very individual battles. You'll meet everyday people like George Biocic, who is learning to do "woman's work" now that his wife Carolyn can no longer handle her domestic duties. You'll read how Mary Baxter's failure to act after her husband's diagnosis left her homeless at eighty years old. You'll meet Dave and Kathy Schissler, who only discovered that Dave's mother was in the late stages of Alzheimer's when she attacked him with a steak knife.

You'll also hear from a financial advisor, a nurse, a nursing home administrator, and a neurologist—all of whom weren't afraid to shed a tear when sharing heartfelt advice that you won't find in any textbook. You may even shed a tear or two yourself, and for that I apologize. The biggest challenge in writing a book about dementia was finding the light in a disease filled with darkness.

While there are moments of levity in the stories that follow, and there's no shortage of love, I admit that this is not a "feel-good" book. As much as I want everything I write to have a happy ending, life isn't always like that. You'll find some of the words here brutally honest, but there's purpose in that:

- I want friends and family members to read what the *real* Alzheimer's is like—not just for the one afflicted with it, but for the caregivers—and to think, "*I had no idea what John or Mary is going through!*"
- I want these words to spur those friends and family members to get more involved. (Generic offers of "*Let me know if I can do anything to help,*" are full of good intentions, but "*Tell me exactly what I can do that will help you the most,*" is far better).
- I want caregivers to find here new ways to alleviate their stress and take better care of themselves, not just their loved ones.
- I want caregivers to read how helpful a support group can be, and then run—not walk—to the nearest meeting.
- I want those same caregivers to know that supported by an organized group or not, they are not the only ones who are going through these challenges . . . that *they are not alone.*

The people in these pages have a wealth of knowledge to share, and knowledge truly is power. In this case, knowledge leads to awareness. The goal of this book is to inform and to educate. Armed with awareness, it's much easier to accept the diagnosis of Alzheimer's and move forward so that all involved can enjoy the best life possible.

It is my sincere hope that the real-life stories you are about to read will give you courage and strength as you step into the world of the *real* Alzheimer's . . . .

1

LIFE GOES ON

THEY SAY THAT LIKE ATTRACTS LIKE. In the case of Bud and Judy Simms, the likeness came in the form of nearly identical Golden Retrievers—both female, and both now ten years old.

"She fell in love with my dog," Bud says. "I brought Leah to the town square, and Judy had her own Golden, Shane."

The couple had known each other for years before the puppy love kicked in, and that's where the likeness gets even more uncanny. They are both seventy-three, and both are from the Midwest. Both raised four children. Bud's wife, Carol, was diagnosed with Alzheimer's ten years before our interview, the same year as the devastating diagnosis of Judy's husband, Chuck. Both Chuck and Carol eventually had to be placed in a home. Chuck died nine years after being diagnosed. Carol died within two months of Chuck.

Judy and Bud know all too well the heartache and trials of being a caregiver to an Alzheimer's patient. Now, as their lives go on without their former spouses, Judy and Bud take care of each other and their two Golden Retrievers.

"Leah, sit down!" Bud scolds as I try to write with a soggy, insistent muzzle nudging my hand.

Leah skulks off and lies down at Judy's feet.

"This house looks a lot better than it did," Judy says. "There were still boxes sitting around up until last week."

Married just over a year, Judy tells how she had to bring in outside help to combine their belongings from two households into one small home. From the looks of things, the decorator has done an excellent job. The walls display four times the paintings as most homes, but they're arranged as artfully as in a gallery.

When asked how they first met, Bud explains that it was five years ago, at an Alzheimer's support group meeting. "I remember the day that Judy came in," he says. "She was a wreck."

Rather than feign indignation, Judy gives a wry smile and says, "That's putting it mildly."

"It was her first day at the group."

"I went in there crying hysterically with these emails in my hand." She waves an invisible sheaf of papers. "I sat down and didn't know a soul, but I was crying my heart out. That's very typical. We get to a point where we just want to go to pieces, and that's when we seek out a group. When you look at that day, and look at me today, I've learned a lot. They thought I wasn't going to make it."

She juts out her chin and flashes a sassy smile. For a woman who started out an emotional wreck, today she confidently leads the very same support group the two are now discussing.

"That day I walked into the meeting with those emails, it was around Christmas," Judy explains. "I always bought presents for all eighteen grandkids. It was a lot of 'doing' for someone who's already a caregiver. I had cut back, but I was still buying, and wrapping, and shipping, which was crazy, but that was just me. I'd bought special things for two grandsons in the service. I had one in Iraq, so I had a deadline with the post office. I said to Chuck, 'Don't touch any of those boxes. I need to wrap the presents.'

"I went out later to where I'd put the boxes and he had gotten rid of all of them. I was tired. When you're a caregiver, you get tired very easily. I had to drive forty miles to find the boxes again, then I got ready to wrap, and now the tape's gone. I'm more frustrated. I just needed to vent the frustration.

"Thinking I could vent to my stepchildren, I got online. The subject line of my email said 'Just venting . . . Another day in the life of Alzheimer's.' I told them the story about the boxes and how frustrated I felt. I sent it to them, as well as to the grandson in Iraq. His mother had told me the week before to share with him everything that was going on at home."

Judy raises her eyebrows. "When they read that email, it got real quiet. Then I got one back from the youngest daughter. Then the oldest one calls, and she had me in tears. 'How could you blame their father for having Alzheimer's?'" Judy mocks.

"Where did it say I was blaming him?" She shakes her head. "I asked my grandson later, 'Did that upset you?' He said, 'No, Grandma, why?'

"That's when I knew I'd have real problems. There's a syndrome out there I call the 'Oldest Daughter Crisis.' We talk about it a lot in the group, because she's the one that's going to give you the biggest problem. There's some connection to dad or mom . . . They want to take over, and they think that because they love their parent, that they know what's best. They think you're not doing it right—that they could do better. It's a real struggle. I finally had to say, 'Look, I've raised four children and I can do this by myself.'"

She explains that she brought up two boys and two girls on her own after an earlier divorce. It was Chuck's children who challenged the way she dealt with their father.

"I sent them all a book about Alzheimer's. I told them, 'After you read this and go to two caregivers' meetings someplace, then we'll talk about your dad's health or the things I'm doing.'"

She glances at a painting on the wall, then looks back. "None of them ever read the book or went to a caregivers group. They knew everything."

I ask Judy if she remembers seeing Bud at the first support group meetings she attended.

"The funny thing is," she says, "when you go in a room with a lot of people, you normally notice the people that are attractive or who catch your attention. When you get in a room with a lot of Alzheimer's caregivers, most of them are looking pretty bad . . . pretty old and stressed. They're downhearted. Bud was just a really pleasant, nice man. He minded his own business."

Bud chimes in. "We saw each other at the meetings, but we weren't paying much attention to each other. She was just another caregiver. I was taking care of my wife and had no interest in anyone. Then, after I put Carol in the nursing home, I was really getting run down. My health was off, my weight was up.

"Carol was in the home for a year and a half, and I started getting more active, physically," he says. "I played golf and I bowled, but it was all just to get my mind off everything. That happens a lot. You don't want to think about it.

"By this time Judy was facilitating the group. I went up to her after a meeting one day and said we should start a group for people whose spouses are placed in homes. When you make the shift from home care to a nursing home, all of a sudden you have new problems, and you're completely alone. Her husband, Chuck, was in Arbor Village nursing home by that time, so I suggested we start a group on Sunday afternoons.

"We got that started," Bud says, "and that's when she fell in love with my dog."

He flashes a smile at Judy. "We were just acquaintances, then I found out that Chuck had passed away. I remembered him, but I didn't know him well. I went to the funeral. As I was leaving, Judy hugged me and told me she was going to California to bury Chuck. I said, 'Maybe when you get back, we'll go to the movies.' We didn't get to the movies for a year, but it all started from there.

"She called me when she got back from California. We met the following night at a local restaurant for hors d'oeuvres and cocktails. We talked for hours. The subject was mainly 'How's your life going?' My wife was still alive. I told Judy I was just looking for a companion. It's a very lonely thing when you go to the town square to listen to the music, and you can't enjoy yourself because you're alone."

He looks at Judy and smiles. "It was a real shock that we connected so quickly after we started dating. I felt guilty about that while Carol was alive, but I knew I'd lost her. When my kids came down, I told them I was so lonely that I had to find a companion." He repeats again that his wife was in a nursing home for a year and a half.

"Once Judy and I started getting more involved, we never called it love. I couldn't say, 'I love you,' because I had a wife."

"He actually stopped me from saying it," Judy says, "So I would just make a noise where the word went." She demonstrates by looking at Bud and saying, "I l-------- you," making a sound deep in her abdomen after the "L."

They laugh softly.

"He knew what I meant," she says. "We didn't feel it was the time to say it, then marriage got in our heads. We had the same idea. We were both seventy-two, and you don't know how long you're going to be here. Why prolong it?" She throws out her hands. "How long do you wait?"

Bud nods. "I always say, 'I started losing my wife ten years earlier,' because you couldn't carry on a conversation. There were times she didn't know who I was. I could have been her dad or her brother. Carol could look at me and think, 'Who is that guy?'"

Bud relates that his four daughters knew what their mother's condition was. Judy's stepchildren had a harder time accepting the changes.

"They don't know what your life is like, missing that affection," Judy says, "or not being able to say, 'Honey, I don't feel good today.' Your partner is gone. They don't reach over and say, 'Why don't you sit down? I'll get you a cup of coffee.'

"You're living with a walking, talking person who has very little emotions left. They're gone to you. You're isolated. If you're young or young-hearted and like to be in a relationship, that's what you're hoping you'll have again in your life. Whether you wait five months, or six months, or ten years, most kids won't be happy, because they've made themselves the one who knows everything."

Judy sits back in her armchair and looks over the tops of her glasses. "The grieving starts the minute you hear the diagnosis."

Bud nods in agreement.

"We know that within ten years, this person is gone," Judy continues. "We're yearning for a real, interactive conversation, and you're living with a shell. But the kids don't understand that.

When they're gone, we're supposed to wait. I was in their lives for twenty-five years. I was the grandmother to their children. I was 'Mom,' but since their father died, now I'm 'Judy.' The oldest daughter doesn't speak to me because I married so soon after their father died. They don't understand that that person is gone to you. It could be ten years!"

Bud talks about his time as a caregiver.

"As I started having to take care of Carol, I did things I swore I'd never do. When I was young, I couldn't change baby diapers, but with Carol I did what I had to do. I learned how to cook. She would try to make a sandwich and wouldn't put anything in the bread. They can only do one thing at a time. They can't connect two thoughts. I could ask her to go in the garage and pick up a bag for me. She'd go to the garage, then forget why she was there. When she dressed herself, she'd have her clothes on, but she'd come out with her bra over her clothes."

"I felt sorry for her, not shocked," he remembers. "The only shock I had was when the doctor said 'Alzheimer's.'"

Judy nods knowingly.

"I decided I had to have support," Bud says. "There were too many questions I didn't know about, so I started going to the support group. I learned an awful lot. The men that don't attend support groups are having a hell of a time. If you're in a group you can cope. You understand it better."

He explains that at the first group he attended, the loved ones attended with the caregivers. "They were talking about all the problems they were having, and I didn't know if Carol understood. I was worried it would hurt her feelings. When she was first diagnosed, I would say, 'Honey, you don't have Alzheimer's; you have *Sometimer's*.'

"I just wanted to get out of there. We stuck it out, but I'd distract her. Then I found another group where the loved ones meet in another room. She didn't want to go to the respite care, but I talked her into it."

Judy jumps in. "The first thing newcomers say when they join a support group is, 'I felt like I was all alone in this.' They don't know the questions to ask. They have thousands of them in their head, but they're so mixed up. They're frustrated and embarrassed."

"Being a caregiver can be a very isolated thing. If you take your loved one out, you worry that they might make a fool out of themselves and you. You go to a McDonald's, and they might order a steak medium-rare. Some people get embarrassed."

Suddenly Bud jumps up from his chair. "Carol, I'm going to be late for my appointment with the dentist!"

"I think you mean 'Judy,'" she corrects him with a laugh.

He laughs back and says, "We both do that all the time."

Bud leans down and gives Judy a quick kiss before heading out the door. She smiles after him, and it is clear that she was right: They didn't need to express their love back when Bud wouldn't let her say the L-word. Their affection is tangible.

Judy settles back into her chair and gives a "What's next" look. This is a woman who has led hundreds of caregivers down the same path she walked for over ten years. I ask her what caregivers need to learn above all else.

"Acceptance," she says without hesitating. "When you're dealing with a loved one who has Alzheimer's, you never know what they're going to do from moment to moment. You're still thinking it's not going to be the way other caregivers tell you it's going to be.

"Some lose the ability to talk. They jabber in syllables. Some haven't talked in years, then all of a sudden something will come out like, 'I like that song.' The day they say something to you that's right on target, your hopes go up that they're going to get better, but it's only for a few minutes. It's good today, then the next day it's horrible. It's the biggest roller coaster ride you'll ever have. You go through the same pain every time that happens.

"It's learning to accept the inevitable," she says. "Your whole life is on hold for this terrible event. Those that accept it and work with it do much better. When things get bad, they know this is just the next step.

"Caregivers who don't accept the changes will procrastinate about doing the paperwork, like getting the finances in order and having a will. We tell them to take care of all that in the early stages. You get to a certain point and you're exhausted and can't think. You cry. You're frustrated. To have to deal with paperwork at that stage is hard. Some of them listen and get things in order. Others, the moment the person dies, they're in the middle of this mess, because they've done nothing and they're not prepared.

"It's hard to do anything once your loved one gets to a certain point. You're tied to your house or that person," she explains. "It gets to where you're physically exhausted, because you have to be there every minute watching what they're doing. They may go in the bathroom and decide to drink mouthwash. They may go in there and not know where the toilet is. A lot of them can't find the bathroom, then when you sit them on the toilet, they don't know what to do. Then they get into diapers and take their diapers off."

Judy explains that the exhaustion is as much emotional as physical. "A lot of caregivers have to deal with people always telling them they should do this or that, or asking why aren't they doing this or that. The biggest thing is the grief . . . not wanting to accept it . . . and the fear, too, of what's coming—of their loved one getting worse, and then death."

She introduces a term she coined to describe the death of a loved one who has suffered for years. "I call it 'blessed relief.' It's a relief for you, and it's a relief for them.

"Many people pray that their loved one will die, and then they feel guilty, but *that is normal!*" She punctuates her words by jabbing at the air, then leans forward and asks, "Would you want to live that way? It's never going to change. Some of the caregivers get it, and some of them don't.

"Caregivers need respite care," she says. "They need a break, to get away from it. They need the kids to step up to the plate, or the loved one's brothers and sisters. When they don't get help, the frustration and anger get worse. You can tell they're having a hard time. Some of these women are perfect, and you see them deteriorating. They lose weight. Their hair is a mess. Their faces are drawn.

"People typically wait too long to place them in homes. It's guilt, because many of them promised that they would never do that. We've been taught that a nursing home is not a good place. In the olden days the homes didn't take good care of people. They were just warehoused.

"We have to be shown that when we put them in a home they're well taken care of. They become part of a family in there. They're socialized all the time instead of having to look at you 24 hours a day. Some of the patients, when their spouses come in to visit, they say, 'Oh, you're here again,' or 'Oh, I have to go play Bingo now.' They have events and activities. The staff keeps them clean and makes sure they have their food. It's amazing.

"It's hard for some people to understand that putting their loved ones in a home is a good thing. They want to spend all day in there with them." She throws both hands out and says, "Why?"

"We have to wean them away. It's not healthy to be there all the time. They need to take a break. Instead, they go in there and get all upset. They say, 'He didn't have a shave today!' And I say, 'Did he shave every day when he was at home?' Then they say, 'But he wasn't neat and clean!' and I say, 'Does he need a tux? Is he going to meet the president?'"

She snickers, but there is a tinge of frustration in the laughter.

"What is the difference? Why do you want to upset this person and force him to have a shower? For what reason?" She sits back and crosses her arms. "Guilt is a real thing. Caregivers need to learn to share what's going on. There are so many who won't tell their friends or neighbors that their partner has Alzheimer's. They decide not to go out socially anymore.

"There's nothing to be ashamed of!" she insists. "You're educating people about this disease by being out in public. Let them see what Alzheimer's is, how it changes your life, and what your needs are. It makes it easier for the rest of us.

"My number-one piece of advice for caregivers is, find yourself a support group. That's the key to getting through it and still being a whole person. I'll lead a group and say, 'Let's talk about sex today.'

They'll open their mouth and look at me like I'm crazy, but they need to understand that everyone's going through that.

"I'll use my husband, Chuck, as an example. I don't think he needed sex at all before the Alzheimer's, but I walked into the dressing area one day and he was standing there with his pants down using my face massager on his private parts! I was blown away, but I didn't want to make a big deal out of it or embarrass him. I knew he was sick, and that was one of the unusual things they do. It would be like scolding a little boy. I knew it was normal, but it was difficult for me. So I just said, 'Why don't you go in the bathroom?' He said, 'Okay'—real easy going. He wasn't embarrassed, because he didn't know it was wrong. If I'd gone in and made a scene, that would have only made him feel bad. They can't help it. They don't have a clue."

She seems completely comfortable discussing the subject.

"Sexuality is a big part of this. The caregivers don't talk about it, but they want to. When I first attended meetings, nobody ever said anything about sexuality, and I was waiting for the topic to come up. So when I took over as facilitator, I started raising the issue on a regular basis. It helps them to talk about it, because they're all in the same boat. If you don't want to talk, you can just listen, but what we say in there stays in there. It's healthy to share.

"Some husbands with Alzheimer's get very sexually motivated. The wives think of them like a dirty old man. I tell them, 'He thinks he's sixteen years old now. What did *you* do at sixteen? Accept that to a point, and learn to deal with it.'"

She talks about the flip side of the issue. "Some have no sexual urge at all. You might want to cuddle, and they don't even know who you are. So you cry, which makes you even lonelier. That's when I tell them that it's okay to have a 'cousin.'" She flashes a cheeky smile.

"Whatever kind of friend you select, it's up to you. You're not hurting them. They're past that. They're not there anymore. It's okay to go out to dinner."

She shrugs her shoulders. "If you don't agree with that, that's okay, too. People come up to me and say, 'Judy . . . .'" She lowers her voice, ducks her head, and mimics them whispering, "'I have a *cousin*.' I say, 'Is that a *kissing* cousin?' They smile and say, 'Yeah,' and I say, 'I'm so glad you have a friend.'"

The coy voice disappears, replaced with firm conviction. "They need to have somebody, some shoulder to cry on. They come up and thank me for bringing it up. It's not uncommon, and it's not wrong. What you do with your friend, that's your business. Some may think it's wrong, but these are the things people need to help them get through it."

Judy tilts her head, then cheerfully announces, "My husband had two wives in the nursing home! One was very flirtatious. She sat next to him all the time and got mad when I would come to visit. It surprised me, but it didn't bother me. That wasn't the Chuck I married anymore, and what part of him was still there had made a friend.

"One night he got his ditty bag and wheeled himself down to her room, and she threw him out! She still chased him all over the place. That's very normal in the homes. Some of the women are very aggressive. They will try to do things, and some succeed. The staff is always watching and trying to discourage it, but things happen. The staff will tell the spouse, because they have a right to know, and that can be a really hard thing for the spouse to deal with.

"There was this one guy in a facility, and his wife bought him some new short pants. She wanted him to try them on for size, so the nurse suggested she take him to a room down the hall. It turns out he had a 'wife' in the nursing home—another Alzheimer's patient—who came in while he was trying on the shorts. She was screaming and hollering, asking the man's real wife what she was doing in that room with her husband with his pants down! Any time the real wife would visit and sit next to him, the other lady would come and push her away.

"You have to laugh," she says. "You have to have a sense of humor. What are you going to do? Accept, accept, accept! It's not easy, but it's the only way to get through it."

She shrugs. "Once you've been through Alzheimer's, I think you can handle anything. I've had a lot of pain in my life, but there is nothing like this. You learn to deal with anything, because you're dealing with the longest death there is."

Her words hang in the air, the laughter from the previous stories dissipating by the second.

"The *real* Alzheimer's is the day-to-day living with it. It's the ugly things and the precious things. It's having to cram the rest of your life together into ten years and hope they're good years. That's why I tell everybody, 'Make good memories. Take them to bed with hot chocolate, and watch TV together. Do something fun. Pretend for the moment that everything's okay.'"

She then repeats what seems to be her personal mantra: "Accept, accept, accept. It's wonderful when you can see caregivers do that. They calm down instead of fighting it."

With that, Judy Simms—a woman who has been-there-and-done-that—throws out a life-saving tidbit to those who are still on their own journey with Alzheimer's. "It's kind of like somebody drowning. The one that fights the lifeguard sinks, but the one that accepts the help gets saved."

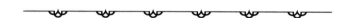

Judy Simms raps on the table. "Okay, everybody, let's get started."

The room is full. Two long tables are lined up end-to-end on all four sides of the room, forming a large square. There are two to three caregivers at each table, and at least half of them continue talking in spite of Judy's raps.

Judy glances at the clock on the far wall. Her lips move upward in a smile, but she is all business as she says, "We have a big group today, so quiet down, please."

This time people listen. All eyes focus on Judy. Some of them look happy to be at an Alzheimer's support group meeting, safe among friends. Others look as if they'd rather be anywhere else.

"I know the holidays were hard for all of us," Judy says to the group. "This is a new year. You're going to be facing some new struggles. I always tell you, take every bit of help you can get—everything to help you get through it—and you will . . . and we'll be there for you."

She nods at the first of two men sitting side by side at the first table to her right. "George, do you want to go first?"

A balding, round-faced man with broad shoulders nods. "Like she said, I'm George." He pauses, then shrugs. "The holiday went okay. The meds seem to be doing their job. The only thing that really troubles me is that if I didn't come here, I wouldn't really know what's going on. It blows my mind how this Alzheimer's takes your skills away. It's hard for me to accept that my wife can't do the things that she was really good at." He shakes his head as if bewildered. "Being here with you guys is a blessing, to be honest with you. I need to learn a lot, because I'm kind of dumb."

The group unanimously protests.

Again George shrugs. "I really have no complaints, but it does trouble me that she can't do the things she was really great at. She don't cook anymore. She don't drive anymore. She don't do all the things that a woman normally does, but she's able to—"

A woman cuts him off from across the room, eliciting much laughter as she shouts, "That's not Alzheimer's! That's finally wising up!"

2

THE GREENHORN

GEORGE AND CAROLYN BIOCIC—which they pronounce "Bye-OH-sick"—announce that they have nothing to hide. They want to use their real names to tell their story. I need to get their permission to do so. I watch as the two of them, dressed in jeans and casual shirts, stand over the kitchen table and read the release form. George takes a pen and fills in both papers, telling his wife that he can't read her writing anymore. He signs his form and shows Carolyn where to sign hers. She lingers a while longer than her husband in doing so, then they both join me in the living room of their cozy villa.

Carolyn is not a particularly petite woman, but she seems small next to her husband. Her hair is dark and curly, framing a sweet, delicate face. She has a childlike innocence about her.

"I'm the oldest of ten," she says. "My father had Alzheimer's, and now I do, too, so my brothers and sisters are all watching me to see . . . ."

George chimes in, "She's donating her brain to the brain bank so all the kids will know the symptoms."

When asked how she is handling the diagnosis, Carolyn's innocence remains. "We're Catholic," she answers, "and I've always said, 'Whatever You send, I accept.' So I guess He must have heard me."

George is anxious to talk about their relationship. "We just celebrated sixty years," he says, then chuckles. "We had our marriage blessed for about the sixtieth time."

Carolyn smiles and sits placidly with her hands crossed in her lap as her husband does most of the talking.

"I was a plumber. She got her RN at forty-five years old, when my last son was out of school. I did construction, then went to work for the city of Chicago. I ended up with a BS, then worked as a superintendent. I retired twenty-four years ago."

He jerks his head in Carolyn's direction. "She made me do that."

"I'm an RN," Carolyn echoes.

George says, "We moved here and there was a problem. She was in denial then, but I guess maybe I was too." He shrugs. "I never dealt with this, so I didn't know. She was getting forgetful. We're talking about five years ago, and she didn't quit driving 'til last year, but let's face it—who knows the symptoms of these things? I think you really accredit it to a 'senior moment,' and you pass it off until something big happens.

"I think she might have blamed me for her situation, so the thing that really got my attention was when she decided to move out of the house. That was a year and a half ago." George jokes, "If you could live with me for sixty years . . . ."

"I blamed everything on him," Carolyn says.

"The leaving was definitely because of the Alzheimer's," he says.

"Why would I leave if it wasn't this?" she asks. "I know that we had a lot of problems, and I guess that was my fault, but he was like a . . . a . . . ."

"A bull in a china shop," George says.

"Yes, that's a good . . . thing . . . ."

She struggles to find the word "analogy."

"Nothing is easy to talk about," she says, leaving one to wonder if she is talking about finding the right word or leaving her husband of sixty years.

"Yeah," George says, "we had a hard time talking to each other. Early on I never spent a lot of time at home. I double-jobbed when the kids were young."

He explains that just before Carolyn left, they had been arguing more than normal. "She would say, 'Whatever is going on with me, you're the cause of it.' She drew money out of the equity thing. Financially, she put a real dent in it. She bought a mobile home close to the church and she bought a car. I didn't know she was buying them. That was eighteen months ago, but she's had the Alzheimer's for five years. The problems were there, but I couldn't say, 'You're a sick lady.' After she moved out, she realized she couldn't cope on her own."

Carolyn nods. "I was there about four months before I realized I couldn't handle it. I had to ask him if I could come back, and he put the rules down."

George ticks off those rules on his fingers: "You gotta get rid of the car, and the mobile home has to go." He remembers, "After she got back, when she told me, 'I can't do this or that,' it was a real shock. I couldn't believe that I had to do it. I was confronted with bills and doing things for her, and I was overwhelmed for a while. For me to serve her was—"

Carolyn interrupts. "I was still doing the cooking, remember?"

He scoffs. "Your skills were gone, hon, believe me. The few things you might have made, it wasn't like you used to make it. There would always be something left out. You were burning stuff. That's when I started looking for support groups. I needed help, and the paper is loaded with announcements about them, but who looks at those things before you need them? Now I'm saying to myself, 'I need somebody to help me.'

"We went to a neurologist, but he kept passing it off as depression, and her situation wasn't changing with his treatments. So we went looking for someone else. There was one doctor in another town that was short-lived, so we were really searching.

"We started going to caregivers' sessions, even though she hadn't been diagnosed. I brought her to the one where they have the respite program, and she said, 'I ain't going back. They're all nuts in there.'"

Carolyn remarks, "The men made jokes, and I didn't like that."

"I'm very comfortable there," George says. "They run a heck of a program. I told the leader, Judy, that the neurologists weren't doing a thing. She recommended this other doctor, so we went to see her. She's an aggressive neurologist. She gave Carolyn all the tests, and she said she was in the early stages of dementia. There's no cure, so we had to bite the bullet.

"She was in denial, but I probably was, too. There's not enough information out there. This is all strange to me. Growing up, all you hear about is things like the March of Dimes and cancer, and all these different maladies. The word isn't out there about Alzheimer's. I'd hear about it if the word was out there, but if you don't read much . . . ." He shakes his head. "I read now more than I've ever read, but the word has to be out there, and nobody is doing that for Alzheimer's people. There's no parades or festivals. There's nobody blowing the horn. It's not *Jerry Lewis and the children*."

Carolyn nods. "There's nothing to help them."

George continues, "But if more people were aware of it, there'd be more people trying to help . . . . Like, Reagan had Alzheimer's. You'd think they'd be using his name. There are just not enough people tooting their horn. You never hear about Alzheimer's. People don't know. I could reflect maybe ten years ago that something was happening to her, but I didn't know."

He turns to look at his wife. "I remember that intersection when we lived in Brandon. We were two blocks from our house and you didn't know which way to turn. So how does anybody prepare when something like that happens?"

Carolyn chimes in, "When I drove all the time, I'd get lost, but I figured, 'Oh, well, I'll pick it up again.' I didn't even think at that time that something was wrong. I figured I went down the wrong road." She looks at her husband. "You wanted me to learn the golf cart, and I kept saying, 'I can't. Why do you think I gave up the car?' I lost my . . . ." She makes a pinched face. "Okay, what did I lose? I lost my . . . the judgment. 'Judgment's' the word. That's why I quit. I figured I'd better stop. I wouldn't want to hurt someone."

"So she's out of denial now," George says. "She gave up driving on her own. Now you ought to see the rug on the passenger's side." He rolls his eyes. "It's creased from her stepping on the brakes. She doesn't like my driving, and I have never had an accident. I tried to make her drive the golf cart, until I heard all the weird stories, like people running off the road, or into the pond, or flipping over."

Carolyn says, "What I did is I went over the bridge on Morse Boulevard in the golf cart."

"She got really uptight," George says, "and I told her, 'Just slow down and you'll be all right,' but she said, 'I can't do this.' I talked her through it, but that was the last time. I just wanted her to try to keep her skills up." He throws his hands out. "I'm not a doctor. I don't' know how to help somebody. I'm trying to use practical stuff.

"So you can't be in denial," he says. "You gotta accept it. I hear that all the time. I listen at the support group meetings, because I'm a greenhorn. But how do you not be in denial? You're afraid of it. I was. She was. Denial is a pistol. How do you say, 'Yeah, you've got something wrong with you'? How do you tell somebody that? And who wants to go to a neurologist?

"So, she gave up cooking. She's not able to put things together. She usually does lunch for herself. She has a power drink or grilled cheese. I do her breakfast or dinner. She won't eat breakfast the way I do it. I make the Irish oatmeal. I do that one day, then I do bacon and eggs and hash browns. On occasions I'd cooked before. Now I do it all, and I don't mind it," he smiles, "'cause I love to eat.

"I have to do all the bookwork, too," he says. "And I never did that. I have yet to balance the bank book, but I'm still liquid." He jerks a thumb in Carolyn's direction. "She would give all the money away. I keep telling her we have to pay the bills. She's a giver, and I have a hard time with that. I don't want to burden our kids. She had seven babies. One passed away at three, so there are six running around. They're all sympathetic. None of them are in denial.

"It's tough," George admits. "I walk away sometimes talking to myself. If I could kick myself in the can, I would, because I don't know what's going on. It's like, *Why is she saying things like this there? Some of them are off the wall!*"

Carolyn looks perplexed. "See, I don't know that."

He looks at her and twists his mouth with resignation. "I know you don't." He turns back to us. "She's gotten to the point where she disagrees with me more than she agrees," he says, "because I have to make all the decisions now, and I ain't the smartest guy in the world."

Carolyn looks at her husband with genuine sympathy. "I should be giving him an easy time now. I think I am, but he gets upset. It's hard on him, and I'm trying to make it easier. I know what's going to happen. I will get to a point where I won't know who I am and what I'm doing. That doesn't frighten me, because I try to accept what's going to happen."

"See, the roles have been reversed," George says, "and I don't know how to do all these things. I was a street guy. I'm not an educated person, but everywhere I went, I succeeded in what I was doing. Even when I went in the army I was the First Sergeant in twenty-one months. I was offered a battlefield commission to Second Lieutenant in Korea, and I said, 'Are you nuts? They're shooting Second Lieutenants every other day!' Now I have to do it all."

Carolyn holds up a finger. "My turn now."

He looks at her, surprised, and allows her to say her piece.

"Am I afraid?" she says. "I know what comes with this now. I don't know how fast it's going to be or how slow. I can't tell, and I don't ask him that."

"Nobody knows," George says.

"So I just take it day by day."

"She's very strong in her faith," he says.

"I know that God is taking care of me," Carolyn announces. "The girls will take me to Mass and we have this big group, so we talk. I learn a lot more about faith and doing what I need to do, and they treat me just like themselves."

"She's not ready for the caregivers' group," George says, but he admits that he is. "It's so helpful because I hear other people's stories, and I'm saying, 'Well, she hasn't done that yet, but I'll be looking for that, and maybe I'll figure out how to handle it.' If I didn't go there with all these things that happen, I would go goofy."

He holds up a finger. "Let me give you an example. How many men did you see at that support group meeting? I'm figuring more men have this disease than women. They're telling stories about their husbands or fathers. I've heard episodes where the men would walk out of the house naked, take the keys, and get lost. Women don't seem to do that. They're not aggressive. So I'm saying to myself, 'Wow, if I had that, I would be a wild man, and you'd have to lock me up.'"

Carolyn nods her head. "That's why when I sat in the room with the people who were worse than me, the girls were saying, 'You aren't there yet, are you?' and I said 'No, I don't like how they talk and how they act.' So I just sit and hope that I'm not the type of person who would try to get out of the house."

"They've got devices where a person can't open the door or drawers," George says. "Like kids. I can't dream of doing that here. I don't hide the keys. She knows where the cash and checkbook is."

Carolyn smiles. "But I can't get in the car to spend it, so . . . ."

George sits back on the sofa and crosses his arms.

Carolyn continues to sit primly. "There's two types of people with this," she says. "There's one that's calm and one that's aggressive. When I see that, I think, 'Oh, my Lord God, I don't want to be like that!' It would put a harder burden on him. I'll just take the slow way."

George shrugs. "I got no complaints, 'cause I'm able to go golfing . . . probably not when I want to go, but I go. She's fine by herself."

"I go in my room," she says. "I have a computer. I stay back there. There's a TV in there. I usually watch EWTN, the Catholic station."

"The problem isn't her personality, so much," says George, "it's her forgetfulness. That's the thing that troubles me, and how I deal with it."

He imitates Carolyn, saying, "'Where's my glasses? Where's the telephone?' Or she covers things up. That blows me away. I think this is a pretty big villa, and it's wide open, but she's got something laying over things. When the phone rings I don't see the light going off."

"I try," she says.

"I know," he admits. "I can't keep track of your glasses. I have enough problems with my own.

"I never knew anybody with Alzheimer's or dementia," George continues, "so all I can say is that this is an insidious disease. It took away all her skills. She had one of the most beautiful handwritings you could ever have, and now she can't hardly sign her own name. She can't really cook, and she can't plan anymore."

"Shopping," Carolyn says.

"I try to do the shopping," he says with a frown.

"He drives me nuts," she says. "He has his own way: 'Now, here's our list, and that's all we can get,'" she mocks. "But I'm to the point that I'll forget to put something down there, and I'll say, 'Well, we'll have to get this.' I know it aggravates him, but I don't do it to aggravate him."

George drops both hands onto the couch. "Well, here's the whole thing: If she needs toothpaste, it takes her ten minutes to figure out, 'Why are all these toothpastes up there? I have to check and see what's in it.' I say, 'Just grab the thing!'

"I never used to go shopping," he says. "It was always just her. Now that I have to go, I don't want to spend any money at all. She says, 'You're a miser,' and I say, 'No, a store's in business to get your money.' My personal bitch is she goes to the beauty parlor to get a permanent, then she's back there a month later, and I say, 'Why do they call it 'permanent'?"

Carolyn lifts her chin. "That, and a manicure, are the only things I can do to make myself feel good."

George shakes his head. "Now it's, 'Write a check for this and that . . . .'

"She was just a great wife and mother, to be honest with you. And she put up with me . . . . That's the whole thing. I'm not easy."

Carolyn reaches over and pats him on the leg. "He's my penance."

He nods. "If I had the Alzheimer's, she'd be in trouble. I'm not a quiet person."

Carolyn's sweet smile is back.

George gives a wry laugh. "I always said, 'If I get goofy, just put me in the car and drop me off at the VA hospital with my discharge papers on me and drive off.'" He crosses his arms and looks at his wife. "And now it's different, isn't it?"

Carolyn Biocic looks back at her husband and nods. "Now," she says with complete innocence, "I can't do that."

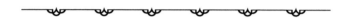

Judy thanks George, then she turns to the man sitting beside him and says, "Dennis?"

All eyes turn to the next caregiver. He wears a crisp blue polo shirt, and his thick, short hair is neatly combed. He leans back, crosses his arms over a broad chest, and says matter-of-factly, "We had a good Christmas. It was different, in that my wife Nancy was there, but not there, you know?"

Several people in the room hum in agreement.

They know.

Dennis neither smiles nor frowns, his emotions well controlled as he continues, "Everyone came to the conclusion that Nancy could get around—with assistance—but she had absolutely no idea of what was going on. Everything is gone."

The newcomers stare like owls. If Dennis' wife is the same age as he is, she can't be much more than sixty-two or sixty-three.

"Like most people, we had some real highlights and some sad moments," he says. "We're very fortunate that we kind of have two more people in our family, and that's our caregivers. I have ladies that come into my house. They come every day. They get her out of bed every morning—even on Christmas morning."

Dennis explains that he hadn't asked for help on Christmas day, but that one of his wife's aides insisted. She had already made plans to celebrate Christmas the night before with her three-year-old daughter.

"I said, 'No, you have to be with your children,' but she said, "No, I'm going to come over at eight o'clock and get Miss Nancy going,' and she did."

There are more appreciative nods, but Dennis isn't finished. "On Christmas Eve, we decided to open presents while my wife was asleep, so it wouldn't be confusing. One of the first things my daughter saw was this envelope on top of the pile of presents. It had our name on it."

He tells about the two loose pages inside—how the same aide who had offered to give up Christmas morning with her family had written a poem for the Humberstone family. "There wasn't a dry eye in the room," Dennis says of himself and his daughters. "She wrote it through my wife's eyes to each of us. It was absolutely amazing."

Judy Simms speaks up. "Tell them how old this woman is."

Dennis laughs. "In maturity, she's probably sixty. In age, she's twenty-two."

There is a universal double-take by those in the room.

"What she wrote ... it was so on target—as if she'd known our family for thirty years." He shakes his head, the cool demeanor momentarily shaken.

"So, overall, it was a great holiday, even though it was kind of like the first Christmas without her. But everybody has accepted the fact that life goes on, and actually, so have I." He smiles now, looking suddenly younger than his years. "I started doing other things."

Judy Simms smiles as Dennis explains, "I went out on New Year's Eve to hear Rocky and the Rollers, and I never thought I'd say it, but I actually had a great time."

3

Early Onset

A LARGE GREEN SEDAN STANDS OUT IN THE DRIVEWAY of the Humberstone residence. The older model car does not quite go with the modern designer home. I wonder if the car belongs to the young caregiver Dennis Humberstone mentioned at the support group meeting.

I ring the bell, and the door is opened by a woman in her early twenties. She is hardly bigger than a yardstick. Her dark black skin is accentuated by a bright, welcoming smile. She wears a uniform consisting of navy blue cotton slacks and a matching print top.

A boisterous beagle jumps at my shins. I pat the dog and introduce myself to the aide. I tell her that I am there to interview Dennis. She seems to know that I was coming.

"This is Molly," she says, looking down at the dog, "and I'm Violet."

In spite of her friendly greeting, there is a gentle shyness about her. Violet welcomes me inside and nods toward the living room.

"I take care of Miss Nancy," she says.

I follow her eyes and stop. I have to take a deep breath. A woman in gray slacks and a neat, white turtleneck slumps on the couch at an awkward angle, halfway between sitting up and lying down. I have been to nursing homes and seen the vacant stares of patients sitting in their wheelchairs, but this is my first encounter in a private home with someone in the throes of late-stage Alzheimer's. It seems suddenly far more personal.

Violet invites me further in and tells me that Dennis will be out in a minute. She slips past me to a second couch placed at a right angle to Nancy's. Both couches face a large flat-screen TV that is tuned to an easy-listening music channel.

"We play the music for Miss Nancy," Violet says, still smiling. "She likes it, and she likes pictures of children and babies, so we have a book we look at together." She nods at a picture book lying open on the coffee table.

Violet seems perfectly at ease. She exudes loving kindness toward me and Nancy.

I feel as if I've entered a foreign country.

Dennis emerges from a back room, smelling of soap. His hair is damp, and he looks a bit startled to see me.

"I just got out of the shower," he says as we shake hands.

I check my watch and see that I'm right on time.

"Where do you want to sit?" he asks, and I choose a table and chairs on the lanai. Dennis takes the far side, leaving me with a view of him across from me, and an equally clear view of his wife through the open doors to my right. I set my tape recorder between us and begin the interview.

"I turned sixty-four on Sunday," Dennis tells me. "Nancy turned sixty-four in September. We've been married for thirty-six years. Nancy was officially diagnosed seven years ago, but the reality is that it might have been a year and a half before that when it started. So, she was actually fifty-seven. She had early onset.

"We have two daughters, one is twenty-nine and the other thirty-four. The older one started a nonprofit foundation to raise money to find a cure for Alzheimer's. She has her big kick-off gala this weekend. There are ideas out there that need initial seed money to get them going."

He explains that only once ideas show merit are people willing to support them with money. Unfortunately, many potentially helpful projects never get off the ground for lack of funding to pursue them.

Bing Crosby croons at top volume from the television set. Dennis seems not to have noticed it earlier, but he now goes to turn it down. Beyond him Violet slowly leads Nancy to the kitchen. Nancy moves like a robot. Not a word passes between her and her husband. She is a far cry from the person he describes when he returns to the table.

"Nancy was a Navy lieutenant when she got out of college. She worked as a physical therapist, treating wounded soldiers coming back from Vietnam. When she finished her tour in Oakland, she got her master's degree in physical therapy and went on to be a professor at a university where we settled down.

"Her employers were unbelievably tolerant," he explains. "When we thought she had Alzheimer's, we signed up for long-term care insurance during the open-enrollment period. To qualify, you had to work at least six months after the date you signed up. Her employers knew what the goal was. Nancy worked six months and five days, so that when we filed the claim, she met the requirements.

"At that point, her job was coordinator of people coming to the university hospital to work on getting their clinical experience— physical therapists, occupational therapists, speech therapists. Did she do a great job? Probably not, but she wasn't treating patients. Now, because of the insurance, we have in-home care seven days a week from eight to four. I pay a little for that, and if I go out in the evening I pay extra, but I'm not complaining."

Dennis discusses when he first suspected something was wrong with Nancy.

"We had a five-bedroom house in Roswell, near Atlanta. We had another house at Lake Lanier, right on the water. For twenty years, between mid-April and mid-September, if people wanted to see us, they went to the lake. Nancy worked three and a half days a week then, so she went to the lake from Thursday afternoon to Sunday evening. One Friday in early August, my daughter Sheila and I both arrived at the same time. We walked in and thought, 'What's that smell?'

"We opened the fridge, and there was a chicken that had gone bad. It was a very noticeable smell. Prior to that, Nancy was meticulous about any little smell, and she said she didn't even notice it. That would be like me watching my sailboat sink and not reacting at all. How did she not know that smell was prevalent? That was the first 'wow' that something was going on.

"My daughter has a master's degree in health policy, and she started doing research on what could cause the sense of smell to go. By Monday evening she was calling and saying that her mother might have some kind of dementia. Sheila immediately set up a doctor's appointment for that Friday. That quickly Nancy and Sheila went, but Sheila wasn't happy with the doctor. They got up and left because the doctor wasn't responsive enough.

"Sheila got an appointment with another doctor, and that one immediately suspected the same thing Sheila did. We started thinking about some of the issues she was having at work, where she was having an unbelievably difficult time getting this complex government report done. That was a big flag. Then we remembered this game we played where you had to say something like 'the Statue of Liberty' and the others would say, 'New York City.' Any time we'd play, Nancy would give it away. We remembered how Nancy used to read all the time, but we noticed she wasn't reading any more. She'd read a little, then forget what she'd read.

"The doctor immediately put her on Aricept and Namenda and scheduled a neurology consult with a scan. At the same time, we got an appointment at an Alzheimer's research clinic nearby. The neurologist and the research clinic thought yes, she had early signs."

Dennis explains that things all started happening rather quickly.

"Our initial attitude was, 'How can this be?' because she had just licked non-Hodgkin's lymphoma. She was never really overly pessimistic. The attitude was, 'We'll lick this, too.' Sheila was ramrodding it—doing the research. Nancy was taking anything that might help. At one point she was taking twenty pills a day and was in a research study that bumped it up to thirty-six pills a day.

"Her diagnosis totally changed everything we thought we were going to do. We went to a class, and they told us, 'If there's anything you're thinking of doing, do it now!' So we put our house in Atlanta for sale. We added on to the house at the lake to make it easier for Nancy later on. Then we bought a house in Port St. Lucie, Florida, because Nancy doesn't like the cold. We had always said we'd retire to Florida. I used to work fifty to sixty hours a week in the corporate world. I was CFO for a Fortune 500 company."

Violet steps onto the lanai and tells Dennis that she is leaving. She lets him know that Miss Nancy has had her dinner. We can see that Nancy is back on the couch. She is sitting up straight, but her head lolls a bit to one side. Dennis thanks Violet, and as she walks away, he confirms that she is the aide who wrote the poem for his family at Christmas.

After Violet leaves the house, Dennis continues with his story.

"Probably the worst time—and the realization that created the most difficulty—was when we told Nancy she couldn't drive anymore. That was pretty early on—six months after she was diagnosed. Many times she would get angry and say, 'I can drive! Why won't you let me drive?' The doctor said that ninety percent of the time she would have no problem driving if it wasn't in congested traffic. From the rural lake she would go around to the park where she could walk, but I knew that if some kid or dog walked out, that would be the ten percent, and she might hit them.

"At one of the classes we went to, a lawyer came in and said that if you've been diagnosed with Alzheimer's and you're in an accident, the other lawyer will go after the patient and all the patient's assets as well as the caregiver and all the caregiver's assets. You could be charged with negligence. We sat as a family—not with Nancy agreeing, but with myself and my daughters—and we agreed that it wasn't the assets, but the fact that if she killed someone, then how would we feel? She never drove from that point on. That was the thing that got the most argument. We're talking about a lady that's fifty-seven, and you're telling her she can't drive anymore.

"She became very frustrated—at times combative." He pauses, then smiles. "There was a point where everyone thought my name was 'GodDamnYouDennis.'

"At the same time, she accepted that these were the cards she'd been dealt, and she had to deal with it. Over the whole time, she never broke down and said, 'Why me?' In some respects she probably dealt with it better than my daughter and I did. We were always focused on finding a cure and how we could make life better for her.

"We put her on different behavior drugs. The doctors made me put all the knives away—not that Nancy would threaten us, but with the Alzheimer's and being unaware, she might. There was a period we felt she was depressed, so we kept all the medicines in a locked cabinet. We were always one step ahead of the things we needed to do."

Molly the Beagle barks from the living room. The little dog is standing in front of Nancy, who is slumped on the couch. She does not respond to the barking.

"It's been a tough time," Dennis says. "It's been rough at every one of the stages up to this point. At each stage you think, 'Can it get any worse?' and it does. Now we're not really husband and wife any more. I'm the nighttime caregiver. She doesn't really know who I am. I had been a very hard-nosed corporate guy. She was the emotional one, and sometimes it just tears me up when we go to the town square. When I sit there watching people our age, and I look out and there are couples dancing who are in their seventies or eighties, I think, 'Wow, how much she would have enjoyed this, and how much I would have enjoyed this with her.'

"So yeah, sometimes it's tough. Very, very tough," he says, gazing off into the yard. "We went down to the square for the lighting of the Christmas tree, and got a good seat. I always explain to people, 'Excuse my wife, she's not being rude. She has late-stage Alzheimer's, and she can't process what's going on.' I never met anyone who wasn't overwhelmingly understanding.

"We were always really big into Christmas, so we went there for the lighting. We enjoyed the entertainment, and they passed around the candles, but I didn't want to light Nancy's candle. She wanted it lit, and people would light it, then she'd blow it out and someone else would light it. So she finally held it for a while, but then she blew it out and was trying to drink the paraffin."

He shakes his head. "You can't just sit there and enjoy things. It's so different when you have to be one hundred percent attentive to what she's doing so she doesn't get hurt. People would come up and say, 'Wow, we know what you're going through. It must be so tough.'"

He snorts. "That would make it even tougher. A couple of times I came close to losing it. I'm doing this by myself—all these things we used to do together all the time.

"People asked me recently, 'What is the thing you miss most?' and it's really just companionship. It's just not there. She's physically here, and she can walk and feed herself, but there's nothing else. Everything has to be done for her."

Dennis explains why he has opted for in-home care instead of placing Nancy in a nursing home. "I feel she's getting better care here." He points to the living room and says, "Someone is no farther away from her than I am now, twenty-four seven. Unless she's sleeping, the aides are right there next to her. Some people have said she'd be better in a home, to get that interaction, but there's no interaction with my wife. There's none. There's just none.

"I think she's happier here," he continues. "In nursing homes, the aides have twelve patients they have to get up and get changed and put in the activity room, so she'd just be sitting in the hall. We have a routine. The aide gets her up, they have breakfast, go for a walk, and she takes a nap. They do some kind of activity, like reading a magazine or drawing something—some kind of interfacing, trying to get her to do something. That's not going to happen one-on-one in a nursing home.

"When her caregiver leaves, I make her dinner and she feeds herself. Sometimes she only eats off one side of her plate so I have to move it around. She doesn't register the left side of the plate, so I have to turn it." He demonstrates by turning an imaginary plate 180 degrees.

"Ninety percent of the time she uses the fork, but she doesn't cut. She starts out with applesauce because we put her pills in it. Then she has dinner, but there's no conversation. She doesn't speak—sometimes gobbledygook. She may say actual words, but we don't understand what she's saying. Then we go to the square for the music."

He explains that the music is the reason they moved here. "When I came to visit a friend here, we stopped at the square, and Nancy was walking around moving to the music. We saw that we could get music three hundred sixty-five days a year here. In the first hundred and twenty days after we moved in, we went to listen to some form of music all but four days.

"We go to the square and she sits down. She doesn't say anything, but I can tell she's enjoying it. We were there last Monday night and she was clapping to the music. She clapped at the end as other people did, so yeah, that's why I go." He nods toward the TV in the living room. "The music . . . the experts have said that music can stay with them a long time."

He finishes describing their daily routine. "We come back from the square around seven-thirty or eight o'clock. We don't leave on a schedule, just when she's had enough. She has ice cream, because she really likes it. She'll eat it and say, 'Ooh that was good,' so I say, 'The hell with it, let her have the ice cream.' These days, if she gets enjoyment out of it, I let her do it.

"I put on a nighttime diaper in addition to her daytime diaper, and she gets in bed between eight-fifteen and eight forty-five. She sleeps through the night and doesn't get up until the aide or I get her up at eight.

"We went through a phase where I had to put alarms on the doors and special handles on the drawers. There've been a lot of stages," he explains. "At times we thought each one was really bad, and now we see those were really good. There was one time that she reached up and grabbed me around the neck while I was driving."

The crazed image is a far cry from the woman who is slowly tilting more and more to the side on the couch. Molly the Beagle sits at her feet and watches her intently.

"I had her in the back seat," he explains, " because she started opening the front door while driving down a four-lane highway."

He crosses his arms. "I don't consider myself smart, but I learn what I have to learn. After I put her in the back seat, she would unhook her seatbelt and grab me around the neck, so we found a device you can put with a seatbelt so they can't unhook it. Then, as a safety precaution, we also got a red band on her seatbelt to put her medical history on in case there was an accident. All of these things you don't think about . . . ."

He sits back and takes a deep breath. "We had great expectations early on. She participated in research studies and memory walks, thinking there was going to be a cure. Then, a year and a half ago, I had lunch with a friend whose wife has Alzheimer's too, and it was like, 'You know what? Our boat has sailed, and now all we can do is do the best we can for our loved ones and make them comfortable.'

"Then it became a matter of accepting it and making the best of every day," he says. "Last year, believe it or not, we spent the whole month of January in Mexico. After we were there, I told our friends, 'This is Nancy's last trip to Mexico. There's no way she can do it again.'"

Molly begins to bark again—loud, rhythmic, attention-getting barks. Nancy makes no reaction, but neither does Dennis.

"The advice I would give someone who's new to this is: Do everything you possibly can early on. Don't wait. When people sit there and say, 'Wow, you sold your house after you lived there for thirty years,' it was no small task. We traveled all over after we moved to Florida. We just did, did, did, did, and did, because people said there'd be a time when we wouldn't be able to do things. In my mind, I didn't believe it would progress to the extent that it has. Now, looking back on it, I'm glad we did all those things."

He purses his lips. "In the last two months, I've come to realize there's life beyond being a caregiver. That's been really important to me. I knew that moving here would be good for Nancy with the music in the town square, but I realized that I was spending all my time taking care of her, and I wasn't taking care of myself. I'd gotten up to almost two hundred and fifty pounds—a combination of not being active and being depressed. I thought that for the rest of my life I was going to be confined as a caregiver to Nancy.

"When we came here, we implemented her long-term care. I got out and was able to do some things. I realized I needed to get in shape. I started jogging and dropped weight. I'm now down below two hundred and ten pounds and I'm going down to a hundred eight-five.   From eight-thirty to four o'clock I'm out doing something. I know there's more beyond the life I had.

"Through the support groups, it's interesting that I see things differently. I went to a group in Port St. Lucie, and one of the guys next to me said, 'I won't be here next week because I'm going on a cruise with my girlfriend.'" Dennis makes a startled face. "I thought, 'You gotta be kidding me!'

"He took me aside and said, "Look, Dennis, I'm not some crazy guy. My wife is in late stage. I met this woman, and . . . ."" Dennis shrugs as his voice drifts off.

"At the time I thought, 'How in the world could you do that?' but since mid-November I've come to the realization that I do everything I possibly can for my wife. That's number one. But after that, what's wrong with doing something for myself?

"I actually went out for the first time last month on New Year's Eve with a woman who lost her husband last year.   I like doing things for other people, and I enjoyed having her come to dinner with a group of us. She was under equal stress."

Now it's Molly, the beagle, who seems stressed. Her barking has become more insistent. She keeps trying to get Nancy's attention, to no avail.

"We got the dog for Nancy," Dennis says. "Molly was her safety blanket. She was so good for her. She's still great, but for the past six months Nancy hasn't even known who she is. A year ago I could have dropped off the face of the earth, and it would have been okay for Nancy, as long as Molly stayed."

Dennis tells Molly that her dinner is coming, and then he gets back to the subject at hand.

"The books about Alzheimer's help you prepare for how to deal with it, and the support groups help, too, but there's not any one 'This is what it is.' There are a lot of similarities from one case to another, but the timeframe of what people with it do, and when they do it, and how they do it—it's different for everyone."

He points at his wife on the couch. "Here we are with Nancy in late, late stage, but yesterday she walked out the door, walked down the hill, and around the block twice with her caregiver. That's a fair walk, but if we went in there right now, held up a pen, and said, 'Nancy, what is this?' she wouldn't have a clue.

"The doctors do this mental test on which you can score 30 points. Early on, Nancy scored twenty-six or twenty-seven out of thirty. For the past two years she scored zero. *Zero.* This is a lady who has a master's degree in medical science. Quite honestly, she was very, very brilliant."

It seems as if the interview is over, but I keep the tape recorder running as we leave the lanai.

Dennis says, "People see me on the square now and they say, 'I thought your wife was late-stage Alzheimer's.' I say, 'Yeah, why don't you go talk to her?' This guy I play pickle ball with went over and talked to her and said, 'Wow. I understand.' Other people say, 'Why are you out with another woman now?'

"If you don't experience it," he says, "people would think that's totally wrong. I say, 'I do all I can for my wife, but I'm a caregiver. She's no longer my wife.' I don't mean that in a negative way. She's gone. Physically, she may be here, but she's gone."

We pass by Nancy, who is slumped over once again in the same position as when I came in.

"Our kids came for the holidays and they said, 'Dad, we're here to visit *you*, because Mom is gone.' One of them said, 'I don't want Mom to not be here anymore, but I don't know how you do it—to be with her, but *not* with her every day.'"

Dennis opens the door for me. It is after five o-clock, and the sound of a live band in the distance drifts on the breeze. The late-model sedan is no longer in the driveway. I know now that the car's owner is, indeed, the young woman who wrote the poem and gave up Christmas morning with her three-year-old for Miss Nancy. Violet will be back in the morning with her bright smile, but for now, Dennis will get his wife ready to go to the square so she can move to the music.

He glances back inside and adds one final thought.

"Statistics say the caregiver has a greater chance of dying before the patient. I'm in the bad statistic zone now. Nancy had some music here today and some interface with the aide, but am I kidding myself about whether that's really a quality of life for her? I don't know. If it was me in her place, I would have no problem saying, 'Please take me to the edge of the cliff so I can jump off.'

"I don't think she would want to live like that, but what will be, will be. We'll make her as comfortable as we can, but that doesn't make it easy."

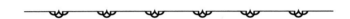

Just down the hall from the weekly meeting, the caregivers' loved ones are enjoying the company of others with Alzheimer's disease. Today they are making crafts with paper, cardboard, and glue, under the guidance of a volunteer. They call this "respite care," for it gives a bit of respite to those who care for them day in and out.

Not all of those present in today's meeting have a loved one in respite care. The next person to speak begins by telling the others, "I lost my husband to Alzheimer's." Then, with a glance at the ceiling, she adds, "Thank God for this group."

Many heads nod.

"My sister has Alzheimer's as well. She's declining very rapidly, especially since daylight savings." She waves a hand. "Oh, God. It was like night and day when we changed the clocks. There wasn't a mean bone in her body

before she got sick, but now she's very angry." She shrugs and says, "So, again, I'm really happy to be here with you people."

Judy Simms thanks her, then turns to the next woman. "Jen?"

"This is my daughter, Beth," Jen says, turning to a younger version of herself at her side. "And now that she's going to be here for a couple of weeks to look after her father, I'm taking off!"

"Good for you!" Judy says.

There are smiles around the room, along with a feeling of relief that one of them is finding some happiness.

"Yesterday I got away, and they did the crossword puzzle together." Jen pats her daughter's arm and says, "She is the best."

"You look good," says a woman two seats down. "More relaxed."

"It's wonderful," Judy says, then turns to a man and woman seated close together. "How about you two? We're all interested to hear your latest—"

Someone interrupts and says, "—escapades!"

The group erupts into laughter.

4

DOUBLE WHAMMY

YOU DON'T HAVE TO ASK PAULA AND TONY FALO WHERE THEY'RE FROM. The minute they start talking, their New York accents take center stage. Actually, Tony was born in Philadelphia, but Paula is quick to point out that New York is where they both spent most of their lives.

Tony is balding and has a prominent Roman nose that speaks of his Italian heritage. Today he sports a pair of golf shorts and a plaid collared shirt. While Paula talks to me from the sofa, he putters about their small house as if he's not listening, but he doesn't wander out of earshot.

Like Tony, Paula is a bit on the short side. Her hair is also short, and white as cotton. She is dressed in white shorts and a green, blue, and white striped top. She wears a crucifix on a chain around her neck. As she speaks, her hands move in concert with her words, revealing mint-green fingernails that are a perfect match with the shade of green on her shirt.

Paula announces that she is only half-Italian, unlike her cousin, Leo, who is the main subject of today's conversation. "Leo was full Italian, just like Tony."

"I'm seventy-eight and Tony is eighty," she says. "Leo was the same age as me when he died last November. We were practically twins. We were born the same month, in the same year, and grew up in the same neighborhood. In our old age, we got very close. As long as he knew who I was, I would be there for him. Once he didn't recognize me, it didn't matter.

"Leo and his wife Alice came to live in The Villages from Barefoot Bay," she explains. "They came to check out the place with seven other couples. We took them around, and they liked what they saw. All seven couples moved here, but at the end, there was nobody anymore. Nobody called, nobody came around. Once they find out about Alzheimer's, people back off."

"They think it's contagious," Tony says from across the room.

"Once they moved here," Paula continues, "we wound up taking them everyplace and doing everything with them. We took them to the casino. We took them everywhere. We did as much as we could for them, because I felt terrible. My cousin had Alzheimer's for three years, and there were people who didn't know it.

"There was another cousin who visited, and she said, 'I want to see Leo and Alice.' She came in and said, 'Hello, Leo, do you remember me?' He said, 'Of course I do! You were a beautiful girl, and now you're a beautiful woman.' She told me later, 'I didn't even know he had Alzheimer's.'

"Looking back to when it all started, we didn't even know there was anything wrong with Leo. We would go driving and he would get confused. I didn't think anything about it."

Tony interjects, "We do the same thing all the time."

Paula goes on, "Then one day Leo took Alice to the shopping mall, and he never came back. We got a call from the neighbor who saw Leo pull up to the house, and he was sitting on the step looking like he didn't know what to do. This was the very first incident. He forgot where he left Alice.

"Leo's brother would never use the word 'Alzheimer's.' He always said 'senior moment.' He said, 'Well, this is what happens when you get old. Everyone forgets.' But this was a big 'forget.'" Paula says. "This was a big one. From then on, Leo didn't get no better. He got worse and worse.

"I said to Leo, 'What do you think is wrong with your memory?' He blamed it on the anesthetic he got in some surgeries he'd had. He said, 'Add up all the surgeries, and I think I lost my mind in all those operations.' So we forgot about it, but little by little he got worse. It was kind of gradual. As his memory got worse, I'd look at Alice and say, 'How's he doing?' and she'd go like this . . . ." Paula points her finger at her head as if it's a gun, and she pulls the trigger.

Tony is unable to stand on the sidelines any longer. He takes a seat on the edge of an armchair across from Paula and joins in. "Leo's wife could not accept the fact that he had Alzheimer's," he says. "If a doctor said something she didn't like, she'd leave the office and say, 'I'm not going back there.'"

Paula makes a sour face. "So then, when we had to find another doctor, she'd say, 'I hope I get one with a name I can spell.' She was very prejudiced. She came from Astoria, in Queens, where Archie Bunker came from. I don't know anybody who's prejudiced like that anymore. She's a dying breed, hopefully."

Paula explains that Leo got to the point where Alice could no longer deny what was happening. "One night we were sitting at the table here eating, and Leo looked at her and said, 'Alice, where's the car?' and she said, 'It's in the garage.' And he said, 'Whose garage?' She told him, 'Ours,' back at their house. So Leo asks, 'How did we get here?' and Alice says, 'Tony picked us up!' Then two minutes would go by, and he'd say, "Where's the car?' Then, 'Where's the car?' You had to be patient.

"Even Tony reached his limit." Paula looks across at her husband, and they share a knowing glance. "We were on a cruise. Thank God it was only five days. Every time Leo walked up to go to the men's room, Tony would go with him. Tony came out of the restroom one day and he said to me, 'If he says one more time *"The pause that refreshes,"* I'm going to throw him overboard.' I said, 'What happened to your patience?'" She laughs, then adds, "He had the most patience of anybody."

"Leo had a good sense of humor," Tony remembers.

Paula nods. "I came into his house one time and I'm carrying a big book with me. It's called *The Nineteenth Wife*, about Brigham Young and the wife he was most devoted to. Leo sees the title, and he goes, 'I always said, if you're gonna *bring* 'em, bring 'em *young!*'" She chuckles. "He was a good three or four years into the Alzheimer's and he could still joke like that."

"Now, Alice," Paula points repeatedly at her own ear, "she was so quiet you had to get her to speak up or read her lips. Not Leo. He was loud, and noisy, and he never shut up."

"Yeah." Tony nods emphatically. "That was Leo."

"Even with Alzheimer's," Paula says, "he was still the same person in the beginning—a talker. But then his brain started to die more and more, and he started not to know. He began to get really, really bad, to the point where we were sitting in the car and I said, 'Will you shut the f— up?!' I didn't say the real word, but I could see his head in front of me shake in surprise. He couldn't believe it. He stopped. He turned around smiling, and he said, 'I love you,' and I said, 'Even though I just told you to shut the f— up?' And he said, 'You wouldn't say that!' He forgot what I said to him in that short a period of time. He just forgot."

Tony jumps in. "The sad part was, I'd be driving, and Leo would be biting his nails." He mimics Leo chewing.

Paula says, "We asked him, 'Why are you biting your nails?' and he'd say, 'Because I'm lost.' He had no more nails left. He was chewing his cuticles."

Paula explains that she and Alice would go to support group meetings together. "At one meeting a man said to me, 'Why do you holler at her so much?' I said, 'She wouldn't be here if I didn't drag her here!' But I wasn't yelling at her. I was poking at her and saying, 'Tell them the truth!' She would say things like, 'Oh, Leo was good yesterday. He washed the clothes.'" Paula makes a sputtering noise with her lips, and says, "He never washed the clothes a day in his life!"

She tells how Tony would sit with Leo and the other loved ones in the respite care room during the meetings. "There was people who sat like this," she says, letting her head loll to the side, "but Leo wasn't like that. He would open the door at a restaurant and say, 'Come ahead, I'm working for tips today.' There were some people said, 'Are you sure he's got Alzheimer's?' and I'd say, 'Yeah, I'm sure.'"

"He was very alert," she continues. "He knew everything. You couldn't fool him. He knew he had Alzheimer's. He would say to

in any way did I even consider that. I thought she was just, you know, overwhelmed with what was going on. I thought she needed some pill or something to perk her up. Her plate was so full with a sick husband and whatnot . . . ."

Paula crosses her arms, then says, "Looking back on it, there was a definite time we knew both of them were sick. One of the grandchildren was having Holy Communion in Palm Bay. We were with Leo and Alice the day before, and we said, 'Have a good time.' Then we thought, 'Oh good, now we won't see them for a whole day," because we were doing everything for them by then.

"Monday, when we saw them, I said, 'Alice, how was the Holy Communion?' She says, 'We never got there. I couldn't find it.' I said, 'You couldn't find Palm Bay?' They were driving around for seven hours and got so hungry that they finally stopped outside of Orlando, which is nowhere near Palm Bay. That's when I said to Tony, 'Something is drastically wrong with Alice. This cannot be.'

"Alice was the driver at the end, and she couldn't drive at all. I wouldn't get in the car with her. She would drive into oncoming traffic."

"She was getting bad," Tony agrees. "Very bad. After a while we would pick them up and take them places, because there was an incident . . . ."

Paula knows exactly which incident he is talking about. She explains, "Alice went to the bank, and she left Leo sitting in the car by himself. When she came back outside, Leo had tried to get out of the car, and was turning blue with the seat belt up around his neck. She ran back in the bank, and they all ran out. She's standing there crying, and they couldn't get that belt off him.

"Luckily," Paula says, "a man came along and got him out. I said, 'Alice, you can't leave him alone.' She couldn't stand the fact that he couldn't do what he used to do. He was a very good husband."

"He did everything for her," Tony says.

"After she was diagnosed, the doctor gave Alice a patch to wear," Paula remembers, "but Alice wouldn't use it. She put it on

Leo. She'd say, 'Oh, isn't it for him?' She was in such denial. She could do denial like I could not even imagine. She said, 'Don't tell my kids. I don't want them to know about me.' They knew about their father, though." Paula tosses back her head. "You'd have to be pretty stupid to be in the same room and not notice something different.

"So when we found out Alice had Alzheimer's, too, I told everybody except their children. I told Leo's brother, his sister, and the neighbors. The family said Alice got Alzheimer's from the morphine when she broke her hip, and I said, 'She didn't know whether she was coming or going *before* she broke her hip!'" Paula throws out her hands.

"I told everybody except their kids, because Alice made me promise not to. Then their daughter Carla came on a visit. They were in the car and Alice was driving. Carla was nodding off, when she felt them go up on the curb. She opened her eyes and said, 'Pull over!' So Alice pulled into oncoming traffic. She went up on an island, and took out two bushes and a bunch of flowers.

"But that wasn't all." Paula flashes her green fingernails. "Carla called me the next day. She said, 'Paula, my parents are fighting. I'm in between them, and they're hitting each other!' I said, 'I'm so glad you're here. This has been going on for a while. Now you seen it with your own eyes, and I want you to tell your two brothers.' And that's how it got back to the children. Carla was there and saw it happen.

"Carla called one time and said, 'I can't get ahold of my parents.' So we went over to their house, and I told them, 'Carla's trying to get you.' And Alice says, 'We answered the phone,' and Leo says, 'Yeah, we did,' but they didn't." Paula shakes her head. "I know he didn't. They were cooking something, and the house was really hot."

"The stuff was boiling over," Tony remembers.

"It was two solid years of taking care of them," says Paula through pursed lips.

"One time in this house he went to the bathroom standing in the TV room," Tony recalls. "He just said, 'Oops, I did something bad.' I helped clean him up, then I cleaned up the rugs. We were always there if they needed something."

Paula explains why Carla couldn't help her parents. "She was thirty-nine years old when she called to say she had ovarian cancer. Leo and Alice didn't know she only had two years to live. From time to time she would call, but she never told them the whole truth.

"When she died, the two of them were sitting there crying. I said, 'If you don't feel like eating, you don't have to,' and Alice said, 'Oh, I could eat.'" Paula snaps her fingers. "She turned it off just like that, and Leo stopped crying, too, because Alice did. They cried, and then they forgot about it, and if you didn't bring it up, everything was fine. So there's some advantage to having Alzheimer's.

"Their son was a contractor building power plants in Iraq," Paula explains. "He would come home, and he was like a whirlwind. He's a real go-getter; he don't sit still for any time. He came home, and when he saw how bad Alice was, he sent her to her brother's place up north. She thought she was just going to visit, and it lasted three months. Before her son placed her, he took her to several nursing homes, but she carried on so loudly that they had to leave."

Tony listens attentively; nodding the whole time Paula speaks.

"After their son got Alice settled, he took Leo to several homes," Paula continues. "Nursing homes are not as bad as they used to be. These were nice. They looked like regular people there, the staff and the patients. Nobody wore pajamas or nurses' uniforms. The first place was really nice, but Leo hauled off and hit a nurse. His son called from Iraq and said, 'Would you go there and check him out?' He had to put his father in another place.

"We went over to visit him in the new place. They told us that Leo was beginning to say sexual innuendos. I knew that Leo wouldn't say any bad words at all, so to claim that he was saying sexual innuendos, it had to be the Alzheimer's. So, this young, beautiful woman comes in to introduce herself. I hear Leo say, 'Oh, you're so pretty. Can I kiss you?' She said, 'No, you're not allowed.' I looked at Leo and said, 'You want to kiss her?' and he said, 'You,

I want to put my tongue down your throat." Paula says this as if it didn't shock her at all.

"I said, 'Not me, I got big teeth!' and I thought, 'If this is sexual innuendo, it's not bad.'

"We couldn't leave that place without him wanting to go home with us. As soon as we walked in, he'd say, 'I don't want to be here. This isn't my house.' I would say to Tony, 'Let's leave, because right now he's occupied and happy.'"

Tony explains that Leo did not die from the Alzheimer's. "He got this thing called 'C. Diff' while he was in the home." C. Diff is a hospital-acquired infection.

"The doctors told us that at any given time thirty percent of the people in hospitals or nursing homes have it," Paula says. "People whose immune system is compromised get it, and they have nothing to fight back with. He died of that four months ago." She twists her mouth. "I didn't go to see him, because he didn't know who anybody was.

"He was only in the nursing home for three months, and Alice missed the whole thing. She didn't see him go down the tubes. When they told her he passed away, she cried like she did for her daughter—for thirty seconds—and then she stopped."

Paula leans back against the sofa cushions. "Their son quit that Iraq thing. Alice lives with him now. He built her a room in his house."

When asked what advice she would give to others about Alzheimer's, Paula does not hesitate. "The earlier you go and get it taken care of, the better. As soon as you notice your memory's getting bad, go to the doctor! Go find out, and take the medicine. It can keep your memory going. The doctors can keep you driving and going to work like a normal human being, but so many people are in denial. 'Oh, so what?'" she mimics. "'I have poor memory. It's no big deal.'"

"Some people are afraid to find out," Tony says. "They need to do more research."

"When the baby boomers are in their seventies, a lot more people are going to have it," Paula proclaims.

"Then they'll put more money into it," says Tony.

Paula crosses her arms. "I think if you examine Alice and Leo and what they did together, you'll get to the bottom of it."

Tony grins. "I tell people it's because they went to the Dollar Store and ate the food from there. I mean, you go to the Dollar Store to buy some wrapping paper and a bow, but I never knew anyone who ate food from the Dollar Store like they did!"

"Alice and Leo were in the same house together," Paula says, pointing a finger, "but they don't know what causes it. Why did she get it, too? They were totally different in their background and their ancestry. They didn't do things together, and yet she comes down with it just like him."

Tony sits forward and says, "We went to a seminar where they talked about what causes Alzheimer's, and I yelled out, 'They ate at the Dollar Store!'"

"Well, you might be right," says Paula, shaking her head. "We don't know . . . but I really got into this, and learned a lot about it, and we got an award from the Martin Luther King group."

Tony gets up from his chair and takes down a wooden plaque from the wall. It reads, "*The Dr. Martin Luther King Jr. Commemorative Committee presents this award to Tony and Paula Falo for outstanding volunteer service in your community, and for your consistent commitment to serve in the hope and spirit of Dr. Martin Luther King Jr.*" The plaque shows one hand shaking another.

"I know some people on the committee," Paula says, "but I didn't know they were thinking of Tony and me. They called me and said, 'You'd better be dressed when you come to the Martin Luther King breakfast,' and I said, 'Dressed? You mean Tony has to wear long pants?' So that's how we found out."

She goes on to describe the event. "They were talking about us taking care of Alzheimer's patients, and Tony started to cry. He thought they were talking about somebody else."

"I just told them what I tell everybody," Tony says. "'Don't abandon them.' They came here with all those friends, and in the end, it was just us."

Paula has run out of things to say. She simply nods. The award speaks for itself.

Tony moves his fingers slowly over the plaque, and says again, "That's what I tell everyone. 'Don't abandon them.'"

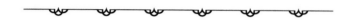

Judy Simms turns to a woman who is attending the support group for the first time. "Okay," she says, "Your turn."

"My husband was diagnosed three years ago," the woman says. "He's very depressed because he's a very sociable person. He has no friends, and I kind of had to tell him the truth why. He's never been in denial. He told all his friends, and now they just don't know what to do. I told him that's why they're not coming anymore. So some folks suggested I bring him here to have him go to respite care."

"Good," Judy says. "He'll feel very important in there. They have a good time."

"I don't know what stage he's in," the woman says, "but he loves to take control of a conversation."

Judy gives an understanding nod. "That's okay, if he enjoys that. Let him do whatever he enjoys."

She points to the next woman at the table. "You're new here, too. Welcome."

The woman appears nervous as she introduces herself. "I'm Mary Ann, and my husband is functioning fine, except I can see it . . . . I've seen it for I don't know how many years. His mother and his sister had Alzheimer's, and he's been in denial since whenever. I remember clearly the morning we went to church, and he put the offering envelope in the plate. Then he started taking envelopes out, and he was going to take them with him. I thought it was kind of funny, and I said, 'What are you doing?' and he said, 'I need more envelopes.'

"There would be things like that once in a while. So he made an appointment with a doctor and they asked him the standard questions. When they gave him the diagnosis, the doctor said, 'Oh, I could tell in five minutes that it's dementia.' My husband said, 'How can you tell?' and the doctor said, 'You cue off your wife.'

"I see it progressing more and more, now, along with the anger. The doctor said, 'You cannot argue with him,' which is why I thought of this group. I was feeling pretty weak, so . . . .'"

Judy opens her arms. "Well, this is the place you need to be. Today we're such a large group, so we're just getting little snippets from everybody, but we'll have a lot for you."

Judy shifts gears and addresses everyone present. "I want to let you know that Dr. Lebron, one of our local neurologists, is coming here to speak to all of us on Wednesday."

A woman to Judy's left blurts out, "Oh! Dr. Lebron is an amazing lady—the way she interacts with her patients."

Judy smiles. "Yes, she's wonderful. You definitely do not want to miss this, so mark your calendars."

5

OBJECTIVITY

TWO MODERN MEDICAL OFFICES face each other along a four-lane Florida highway. The parking lot between them is empty—the patients who earlier parked there are most likely eating dinner at this hour. Behind the medical building on the right, in a spot reserved for staff only, a car sits with its hood up. A woman in colorful nurse's scrubs leans over the engine and frowns. A man comes out of an unmarked door with a battery charger trailing a power cord. He leans under the hood beside the nurse.

Behind them emerges a short, olive-skinned woman in denim Capri pants and a sleeveless, blue floral top. Her burgundy-reddish hair is cut in a short bob. She stands back and observes silently as the man applies life support to the battery. Seemingly satisfied that the patient will survive, Dr. Maria Lebron turns to go back into the building. Looking my way, she stops, and motions for me to follow.

We pass through a staff break room and walk down a hall past several exam rooms. Dr. Lebron's steps are heavy and her shoulders sag. "My nurse was out today with a stomach upset," she explains with a thick Hispanic accent. "I was on my own all day."

We walk through a doorway and emerge into a large, empty waiting room. The doctor crosses to the side with windows and sinks into a padded armchair.

"What can I tell you?" she asks. Smiling seems to take an effort after her long day.

I ask what the most difficult challenge is for her Alzheimer's patients.

She thinks for a moment, then answers, "It is the disparity of roles that creates a big stress for couples. That's what I see every day. The problem is the relationship between a husband and wife. It has to do with who has been in charge to that point," she says, meaning that one person usually plays a dominant role.

"That makes the whole difference: Who is in charge in your marriage? Who does the finances? Who makes the major decisions in the house? How do they make them? These people that are developing Alzheimer's now, most of them are seventy-plus in age. The relationship between husband and wife of that era is totally different from my era," she says, speaking from her viewpoint in her early fifties.

"Most of the time the husband is in charge," she continues. "The wife is a secondary element in the house. She may know about the house, but she doesn't know about the rest."

She shakes her head. "I have had a lot of patients where if he's the one that has the Alzheimer's, she doesn't know what to do. And it's not about the disease—they don't know what to do with the *life*."

If her wording at times seems awkward, it is only because English is her second language. Dr. Lebron is not the slightest bit awkward when expressing her opinions.

"That is one of the problems that I see day in and day out," she repeats. "They don't know what to do. They have no idea how to handle the house, a repair, buying or selling a car, where to move. They are not capable of making decisions independently, and if the wife is the one who has Alzheimer's and the husband is used to being the man of the house, he doesn't know how to handle all of the domestic chores.

"So they are dealing with a lot of stress. Sometimes I look at them, and you look into empty eyes on both of them. Forget about the Alzheimer's patient!" she says with a flip of her hand. "I get a lot of them in the early stage, so it's not like they come with this empty, blank stare. It's the look on the face of the caretaker, who doesn't know how to handle it.

"So, what do I do? I tell them exactly what to do. I go one, by one, by one, by one." She counts on her fingers, then mimics herself talking to her patients: 'These are the needs. This is what you've gotta do. You have to check your finances. If you can't do it, you've got to find someone who can help you with that.

"Ah . . . ." She gives a small jerk, as if a new thought has just occurred to her. "Then there's the *other* problem," she says, "the relationship between father, mother, and children."

She inhales slowly and considers her words before elaborating. "There are a lot of couples that have very close relationships with their children, and they can rely on those children for advice and support, but there is a big group that can't. American culture is so different from mine. I am Puerto Rican. I came here at age 32, and it was shocking.

"There's a problem in the family nucleus in this country. There's no problem until you get old. Kids have to understand they're part of the family for life. That's the way I grew up. Family helps each other. We're always there. For example, my mother lives with me. She has been in my house for the last ten years, and it is perfectly fine. But that's like *unseen* in this country. You don't see this. With the computer and Internet, the children are disassociating even more. I don't know what's going to happen.

"To the children of someone with Alzheimer's," she says now, as if addressing them herself, "your parents need help. You need to be involved in the economical and emotional aspects of your parents' lives. You need to know what their finances are, what they want for themselves as they grow old. You need to discuss this with them.

"Ask your parents, 'What would you like to happen if you get Alzheimer's? What would be best for you? Do you want to stay in the house? What economic resources do you have?' But what I see every day, is first of all, people don't want to give up independence, which I do understand. But when you have a couple of people where they are both medically ill—or where one is medically ill and the other is mentally ill—you need to be objective. Objectivity is so important. You have to protect that couple. It's very difficult for caregivers to be objective.

"Over and over I have to sit down with my patients and tell them: 'You have high blood pressure, you have diabetes, you have difficulties with your heart. He has dementia. If anything happens to you in the middle of the night, who is going to help? Who is going to come and take care of him or her? Who's going to give him the medications? Who's going to take care of the cooking? Who's going to take him to the doctor while you're in the hospital? If it happens overnight, is there a person or is there a phone number you can call and somebody's going to be here to take care of that person?'

"It's as simple as that!" she says, throwing out her hands.

"'Well, I have my kids . . . ' she says in a higher voice, mimicking a typical patient's response. "Well, your kids are up north! They can have all the good intentions, but it could take them 48 hours to come down here, and they have a job, and they have to get a ticket on a plane at the last minute to run here, when you should address this beforehand! That would give them enough time to assess the situation, to get on a plane, to make arrangements, and get here.

"You have to have that in place, but they say to me, 'I'm fine. If something happens to me they'll take care of him . . . .'

"No!" She is adamant. "Don't leave it to chance! It's not fair to that person, because you could just—" Her voice suddenly becomes barely audible as she whispers, "—*drop dead* . . .

". . . and what's going to happen to the other one?" she asks now at a normal volume.

"Make plans! Make plans! Make plans!" she says, karate-chopping her left hand with her right. "I cannot say it frequently enough. I don't know how many times a week I say that. 'Make plans ahead!' If your kids are in a bad economic situation, they're not going to be able to jump on a plane and come. They're not going to be able to physically help you. I have had those situations. Find a place where you can all live nearby, but don't wait until the last minute. And they do." She shudders. "Oh, God, yes, they do.

"I have been able to convince a lot of people along the way, because I preach this constantly—*constantly*—to my patients. 'Make plans ahead. Don't wait to the last minute.' For me that's so important, to have a say in these things. I've lived through it with my mom, and it's very difficult. I'm not preaching something that I haven't lived. I know this is possible. You need to accept your age and your limitations and take care of things.

"It gives you more integrity if you, as a person with Alzheimer's, go with your partner and choose—make a decision—of where you want to be—what kind of place you want to end up in. Bring in the family. Decide which place you want to be at the end. Sometimes the kids want to take a parent to their house in a different state. The problem is, by doing that you may be uprooting them from friends and activities. They would be too isolated. So you have to think of different aspects of moving.

"It's not as simple as you just put them in a nursing home. They have to look for other choices before it gets to that. I'm a strong believer in having help in the house for as long as possible. A patient with Alzheimer's is always going to feel better and respond better when they are in the home.

"The problem is, the caretaker cannot do it twenty-four seven. They cannot, because they will burn out. It all depends on how long they can pay for help in the house, or get family and friends to help. The caretaker should get out and forget about that loved one for a while, because you have to take care of yourself. If you're depressed or anxious, go to the doctor and take a medication. If you're tired, get somebody to take care of him while you go get rest for a week.

"Don't think you're the only one who can do it, because it's not true. There are a lot of lovely people that help, and they do it very nicely. Eighty percent of the time the patient feels relaxed with somebody else. They're okay," she says with a wave of the hand. "They get a break from that caretaker.

"You, as a caretaker, you're nagging at that person. And you're going to do it, so it's okay to feel guilty. Sit down, cry a little bit, take a deep breath, and go back and change the behavior. You are going to nag. Just realize why you're doing it. It's usually because they're doing something that's annoying you, and they can't help it.

"The person that has the disease doesn't understand why the other is nagging. The caregiver doesn't understand why he doesn't react to what she's saying and it's like—" She knocks her knuckles together. "There's an impasse right there. And that's what I think is the worst part of the disease: when this person is just not capable anymore to be your partner—a cognitive, able partner. That is when everything comes to a stop. The problem for the caregiver is that they have the emotional charge of seeing their loved one . . . ." Her voice falters and her eyes fill with tears.

"Losing that partner is very sad. You have to live through it to understand. It's very sad. It's somebody you share memories with, and everyday life, and TV programs, and jokes, and that starts going away. You don't have that anymore. You now have a child that you take care of. And you have to tell that child what to do and what not to do, because they forget to do the things they did on a regular basis, things as simple as turning on a TV with a remote. They can't do it. They see the remote, and they don't know how it functions. They don't know how to use the phone for a call, how to shave," she says, running an imaginary razor over her cheek, "or how to put on a shirt—which side goes up or down, how to button—things that are so simple.

"At the beginning it's not that bad, but as time goes by . . . ." She lets out a big sigh. "They need to be patient, and that's hard." Then, as if someone might hear her in the empty waiting room, she mouths the words, *And that's the problem.*

In a normal voice she advises, "Number one, you have to understand what's going on in their brain. You have to forget who they were, and treat them for who they are now. That's something that I see every day with the caregivers. They try to address the person like they were before. They try to get them to make decisions with them. They ask for their opinions, and I'm like—," she pulls in her chin and makes an *Oh-my-God* face.

I point out that she is gripping the arms of her chair, and she replies, "Yeah, I do this a lot."

She puts her hands back in her lap with deliberate daintiness. "Well, you know," she says now in the kind of soothing voice that she would use with a caregiver in this situation, "he just cannot completely understand what we're saying, so we need to *help* him make that decision . . . ."

I comment that it sounds as if she does a lot of educating the caregivers in how to deal with this changing person. She sits up and throws out her hands.

"That's it! It's like having a child again! The problem is, with a child you're teaching, and with this adult-child, you have to do things for them. It takes patience and acceptance. That's not your partner anymore. That's not your father anymore. This is one of the things I see over, and over, and over. They try to deal with the person as if that person doesn't have a problem. They think that is the best way to treat them, and yes, you have to talk with them, and you have to make them part of the plan, but at the end of the day, you have to make the decision that is best for them.

"You have to tell them, 'Well, we're gonna do things this way, because I think this is going to be better for you and me.' You do this whether he understands or not. Whether he likes it or not is irrelevant. You've got to make the decision that is best. You explain, and you try to be nice, and you have to be understanding, and sweet, and polite, but at the end of the day, *you've got to do it!*" She emphasizes each word. "Don't sit and wait!"

She smiles extra sweetly now and says, "And they sit and wait. And I ask what they're waiting for, and they say . . . ." She leaves the answer hanging for a moment, then whispers, "*A miracle.*"

Her face shows that she takes none of this lightly. I ask how she can deal with the emotional turmoil her patients face day in and day out.

Her answer is matter-of-fact. "Because I love what I do. Just being able to sit with a couple . . . to see a father and daughter, a mother and son, and being able to help them through it . . . that keeps you going. I treat them nicely—like people. That's it. I talk to them. I am open. I am honest with them. I try to understand their problems. I try to address the different problems of each one of them. And I love them. I really do. I don't think that being a physician is just giving you a diagnosis and a prescription. Anybody can do that.

"I develop a relationship with my patients. I have had people who are absolutely delightful. I mean *de-lightful*. I have two patients that I have been following probably for ten years. They're in their mid-eighties now, and they are sweet. I met them when they were still talking, and they are ten years down the road now and talk without sense. They can't make a whole sentence that makes sense, but they are still the same wonderful persons.

"Now, number one, their personality was very kind to begin with, and number two, they had big family support. One of them has three or four boys. They have taken him on vacation. They love to do picnics with him. They allow him to do as much as he can, and there is always this love, and care, and support from the sons, the in-laws, and the grandkids. They take turns as far as where he's going, who he's going with, and what he's going to do.

"It's the same thing with the other gentleman. They only have one daughter, and every Saturday she comes and sits with her father the whole day. Every summer they go to a beach house and spend it together. They have been so good about it. It does make a difference because you can see . . . I don't have to give them any type of medication for behavioral problems. They get up, they eat, they sleep . . . they're happy. They don't have a memory. They can't dress themselves without help. One of them can't feed himself. The bottom line is: family is all."

A door on the far side of the waiting room opens. A tall man with thick salt-and-pepper hair steps in from the hallway, and Dr. Lebron's eyes light up.

"Hi, darling," she says. "Are you just finishing?"

"Yes, baby," he says. "I'll meet you at home."

"Okay, bebé," she says, then turns to me and introduces her husband, a physician who has his practice in the same building. It is well past most people's dinnertime.

Her husband departs, and in the ensuing pause, I ask Dr. Lebron if there is any subject we haven't touched on.

She thinks for a moment, then answers simply, "Yes. Sex." She rolls her eyes and says, "Oh, God, it is a very touchy subject. You have to figure out, what does the couple want? If he's hypersexual to the point where he's being promiscuous, you know that is a behavioral problem that has to do with the disease. You have to manage that with medication, because that's not healthy for the patient or the caretaker.

"It's not a matter of having sex—it's the promiscuity. They can attack caregivers. That, you have to treat. It has to do with frontal lobe inhibition. The frontal lobe gets damaged, and they don't have the ability to control those impulses. There are certain types of dementia where this is more common.

"So, sex . . . . If you had a healthy sexual relationship before, and he is capable and you are capable, then keep going. If there was none before, and now he's getting hypersexual, you have to tame that down. I mean, you have a wife that's 78 years old that has backaches and you haven't had sex in ten years . . . ." She laughs, then concludes, "Yeah . . . there's nothing wrong with having sex, but it has to be addressed according to that couple. They shouldn't feel bad about discussing that. It's part of life.

"You have to accept the disease for what it is, and try to do the best with your life with what you have, instead of being afraid, and depressed, or mad . . . no!" she almost shouts. "Just take it! Understand it, and live the best you can with it. That's what you have to do.

"If you can accept that that's going to happen, and you prepare yourself ahead of time, when you get to that point, you have already worked it out to a place where the changes don't affect you as much. I'm not going to say that there aren't going to be bumps along the road, but if you accept it today, those bumps are going to be very small and much easier to go over.

"If I don't help the caretaker to accept this and change, I don't do anything good for my patients, because what else do I do?" she asks. "Give them a pill? Evaluate the stage of their disease, and tell the caretaker, 'Well, this is what it is'?

"Unfortunately," she admits, "from a medical standpoint, that's all I can do right now. I don't think we're going to see a cure for Alzheimer's anytime soon." She shakes her head with this gloomy pronouncement. "I don't know . . . maybe I'm a little too objective sometimes. I don't think we're going to see a cure anytime soon because of the way the disease works, and what it does, and how it does it. I don't believe in false hope, but only God knows.

"There are several different types of dementias," she explains, "and what triggers that change is basically part of growing old. I think we're going to have more medications. That I do believe. They will slow the progress even more. That's what I see. What I see coming down the pike is medications, because what they're doing is they're looking at the different aspects of the physiopathology of the disease.

"Up to today, we only had one group of medications. There are different names, but they have the same mechanism of action. Then the drug Namenda came along. That's a different mechanism of action. Now all the medications they are working on, and all the research that they're doing, is in a completely different place—it's to try to work on all of these metabolic abnormalities that are causing the accumulation of all of these things in the brain."

She waves a hand and says, "I don't want to talk medical, but that is going to reduce even more the progression of the disease, because you can actually block that at the very beginning. So, first of all, we need a better way of diagnosis. And that is one of the problems. That's something that I have a major problem with. Up to today the diagnosis of the disease is based on patients that are already in a mild to moderate stage. At that point, what the hell am I giving you?" She throws her hands out in frustration.

"If we can get you diagnosed a little bit earlier, we can slow things down."

"What happens today is you may have a bit of memory problem. That is called, 'Mild Cognitive Impairment,' and there is no treatment for MCI. The book says that fifty percent of those patients are going to progress toward Alzheimer's. Do you want to be the one taking the chance and not getting treatment?

"So I think they are going to be able to link MCI with findings in the brain. That's what we need to do. That is going to make the general population of physicians able to identify those cases and start them on treatment, and the earlier the better. By putting them on medication early, you are giving back to that person a lot of good years."

She uses data to prove her point: "If you leave Alzheimer's untreated, what you're going to see is five fair years, three bad, and two terrible.[1] But if you can treat it early and get eight good years, ahhhhh!" She smiles, tilts her head, and points a finger. "Then, by the time you start getting into real trouble, you're going to be so old and decrepit that you'll be too old for any major concern. After that, anything that happens is okay. You can take it," she laughs, then grows serious again.

"I just want to help people. We need to get more awareness of the disease instead of being afraid of it. People need to understand that they need to treat it as early as possible. As I said, there are currently only two different groups of meds, and that's it. That's the main problem we have. They slow the progression of the disease. That's why in accepting the disease, taking the medication as early as possible, you are really slowing the progress a lot. *A lot.* And hopefully, I would say, in five years, we will have at least two more groups of medication.

"So, yes, accept what the person has. Embrace it. Learn about it, and do as much as you can with it. Don't be afraid of it and just sit in a chair. Some people just enclose themselves." She clarifies that she is talking about both the caregiver and the patient.

"If you make the diagnosis in an early stage, that patient is ca-

---

1   According to Dr. Amanda G. Smith, M.D., Medical Director, USF Health Alzheimer's Center: The average time from diagnosis to death has traditionally been eight to ten years. However, with (and even without) treatment, this can vary greatly. Some people decline rapidly over two to three years, and some decline at a snail's pace over twenty. Nevertheless, early treatment is crucial to slow down the decline in memory and function, and decrease the frequency and intensity of behavioral problems, which can arise in up to ninety percent of patients at some point in their illness.

pable of understanding most of what you're talking about. He or she is at a point then to make decisions and take charge of it. And it is talking about it—not being afraid of it, and making the decisions ahead of time—that makes all the difference. Talk to your family!" she says with animation. "Talk to your friends! Discuss it!"

After a long, hard day at work, it is talking about her patients—discussing her passion—that has brought Dr. Lebron back to life. She looks around the waiting room that will be filled again the next morning and gives a knowing nod. "My patients with Alzheimer's are very frightened. Some of them understand what's happening, and they can see it. Others don't understand, and they are frightened of any change. You can see the fear either way."

I ask if there is any way to ease that. She lowers her head as well as her voice as she says slowly, "Love . . . understanding . . . and compassion." She sticks out her thumb and points it toward the ceiling. "Last time I checked, that's what He said."

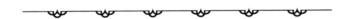

Judy nods at a woman with dirty-blond hair seated in a chair along the back wall. "Okay, Jackie?"

The woman has a defiant look. Her jaw is set, her eyes slightly squinted. "Hi. My name is Jackie Campbell, and I'm not going to cry, so I'm going to be brief."

She has a deep voice, devoid of emotion. She speaks rapidly, as if spitting bullets.

"My husband passed away December fifteenth. It was a nightmare, and someday we'll talk about it, but right now, I just . . . ." Her voice drifts off, and for a moment there is a crack in the veneer, then she squares her shoulders and spits out the rest.

"I think most people know what I went through. It's an awful, horrible, terrible disease . . . a terrible disease.

And I loved Biff to death, but he's in a better place, so . . ." she shrugs her shoulders. "So that's me."

That's Jackie Campbell.

She shakes a dismissive hand and barks at Judy, "Go."

And Judy Simms moves on to the next caregiver.

6

THEY SHOOT HORSES, DON'T THEY?

THE SIGN HANGING FROM THE LAMPPOST in the front yard reads "Biff and Jackie Campbell." A front door isn't visible. I cautiously step through a screen door onto an enclosed lanai and find two more doors. I knock on door number one, and as I wait for someone to answer, I notice a framed eight-by-ten photo straight out of *Secretariat*. In it, a jockey is holding the reins of a sleek, brown thoroughbred. Several smiling people stand in front of the horse—smiling, no doubt, because of the seven thousand dollar purse indicated by a small plaque at the bottom of the photo.

In the picture stands a trim woman with a full head of blond hair, and I recognize her as a younger version of the woman I've come to interview. I met Jackie Campbell briefly at a caregivers' support group meeting, and although the photo is a bit faded, she has the same spark I first saw there. I look at the man beside her in the picture, and am wondering if he's her husband, Biff, when door number two opens to my left.

"Some watchdog this is," Jackie says by way of greeting. She nods her head at a white and tan furball running in circles at her feet.

I cross the lanai and as I step inside, Jackie tells me the dog is a Maltese-Lhasa mix. She shakes her head with what seems like feigned disapproval. "He didn't even let me know you were here."

We trade greetings and small talk as Jackie leads me through the small, tidy house to a dinette set in the kitchen. I smile at the plate of goodies on the table. It's a thoughtful touch.

"Go ahead," she says, following my gaze. "They're all home-made."

I thank her as I bypass the cookies for a piece of cinnamon coffee cake. My hostess seems appalled when I decline a cup of coffee. She pulls her own mug out of the microwave and comments that she lives on the stuff.

Jackie takes a seat across the table. She looks tired, and apologizes for her hair. It's a bit disheveled, but nothing else about her is. The dark eyeliner around her upper and lower lids shows that in spite of the stress she's been under, she still takes some time for herself. Her eyes have that same spark I noticed the first time I saw her. Actually, it's not so much a spark as a steely glint. She's friendly, to be sure, but there's something about that spark that says you might not want to cross Jackie Campbell.

The house is quiet—almost *too* quiet. Biff has only been gone for forty days.

"We were married forty-seven years," Jackie says. "We met at a club in Baltimore. I worked for IBM in computers, and I worked for Spiro Agnew."

I want to know more about this unusual connection, but she's off and running about Biff.

"He was a blacksmith, a horseshoer. He went to all the race-tracks in New Jersey, Miami, and New York, and he shod the horses."

I flash back to the photo on the lanai while Jackie holds up a finger. "That's s-h-o-d," she says, stressing the "D." "I tell people that, and they think he *shot* horses. He didn't shoot horses."

We laugh and she takes a sip of coffee before going on.

"We lived in Bellaire, Maryland, then we moved outside Atlantic City, because he worked the Garden State, Atlantic City, and Monmouth Park circuit."

This explains the accent.

"Our son died ten years ago of a massive heart attack at twenty-nine," she says, and the air seems to go out of the room.

"So we sold everything and came down here," she continues. "It was a tragedy. It was just awful. I honestly think that's what triggered the Alzheimer's in Biff. He thought the sun rose and set on that boy. Rhodes was the athlete Biff always wanted to be. Biff was five-foot-nine and a hundred and sixty pounds. Rhodes was six-feet and weighed two hundred and ten. I noticed a few strange things with Biff after that, but I never made the connection until the incident with the phone."

I ask her to explain.

"It was four years ago. My daughter Buffy was here, and Biff was sitting right there." She points to the empty chair to my left. "The phone rang, and Buffy said, 'Aren't you going to get that?' and Biff said, 'I can't.'"

Jackie shakes her head, remembering. "We were like, 'What do you mean? It's right there!'"

She points to a wall phone that's no more than three feet away. From where he was sitting, Biff would have only had to reach up and grab the receiver.

"Then he had a flip-out. He got very hostile . . . angry. He said, 'If you want to answer the damn phone, answer it yourself!'"

Jackie explains that Biff did have a temper, but his reaction that day was unusual. "I'm like, *What the heck was that?* That was very rude and nasty, but he blew it off, like nothing was wrong. He said he just didn't feel like answering, but he never answered the phone much after that. He couldn't communicate that way. The last two years with the Alzheimer's he couldn't speak. Syllables came out, but not words, so on the phone, someone talking in his ear didn't register."

Jackie tells of a later incident at a horse farm where Biff went back to work. She noticed that the writing in the ledger where he recorded the horses he'd shod was too neat. When confronted, Biff admitted that he was getting the lady in the office to write in his daybook.

"That was a flag," Jackie says. "I sent him to the VA hospital, and he talked to a psychologist. They blamed all the problems on the death of his son. They diagnosed him as depressed."

A bout with prostate cancer and subsequent surgery left Biff's faculties further impaired. Jackie blames it on the anesthesia. "Any

√ time a person with Alzheimer's is sedated, their abilities never come back. I've learned all this since."

It was another year before a visit to a neurologist.

"The doctor said to draw a box inside another box, and he didn't know what that was. She said to write a sentence, and he was embarrassed. He couldn't do it. There were supposed to be two days of tests, and at the end of the first day I said, 'What time do you want us tomorrow?' and she said, 'No, it's over.' He was already in the late stages.

"Three years ago we were driving back to Florida on I-95 from our other home in New Jersey, and I didn't think there was a problem. We always got off the highway at mile marker 95 in North Carolina—our halfway point. Biff said we'd passed our exit and I said no, we were at 89. He said the numbers went the other way. He didn't get it, and I could see that he'd panicked. We finally got to the hotel that night and I said, 'Biff, this isn't good. You were very upset, and I think I should drive the rest of the way.'

"When we got home I said, 'Biff, do you know you've been diagnosed with Alzheimer's, and if you have an accident, we would lose everything you've worked your whole life to attain? Would you want that?' He said no. He never drove again, and he never bucked me. I'm a strong personality, and he knew I meant it. We didn't argue that much. We had tons of fun. We traveled a lot and did a lot, but after that I did all the driving and all the paperwork."

I ask how she got involved in the support group.

"I go to the church where they have the meetings," she says. "The minister made a statement in his sermon one day about Alzheimer's and the group, and I started going. I learned a tremendous amount. Everybody should belong to a support group, and I'll tell you why." She leans in and taps her finger on the table. "I call it a bitch session. When I go to that group, I'll say, 'Can you believe my husband did this or that?' and someone else says, 'Oh, yeah, my husband did that two years ago.' So it taught me what to expect.

"I remember the first time Biff had an accident. He had messed himself, and that was unbelievable. This was a very strong, virile man, and I had to clean him." She rears back in her chair, makes a face, and shakes her head as if to clear the memory.

"But that's the kind of thing I could say in that group. I told them what happened and I said, 'I can't stand smelling it! It makes me sick!' And one of the women said I should use Campho-Phe-nique. I thought I was supposed to put it under his nose. I asked 'How is that going to help clean him?' They all roared with laughter, and said, 'No! It's for you! You put it under *your* nose so it doesn't smell!'

"They teased me about that forever, but we all say, 'What's said in this group, stays in this group.' It's those kind of things that when I go back now and see people in the mild stage, I can say, 'Oh yeah, I got a hot flash for you. You have to take over the person's entire life.'

"We feel comfortable at the meetings. I'm a speak-out kind of person, so one day I went and I was really frustrated. It's very trau-matic dealing with an Alzheimer's patient." She runs both hands across her scalp, then makes two tight fists and pulls her hair. "I said to them, 'I hate him!'"

She sits back, smoothes her hair, and explains, "I love him dearly, but I could vent to them and they didn't judge me. That's very important.

"Yesterday a friend said to me that all she could think about was the time I said to her, 'I hate him. I don't think I can do this anymore.' This woman has been my friend for fifty years, and I said, 'You should have walked in my shoes. I never hated him.'" I was frustrated, like the time he peed on the floor. But see—there's the difference. If you said that to the support group, they'd never throw it back in your face.

"There was a lady I sat next to in the group, and she said about her husband, 'I can't stand him. I can't go on with it.' And we talked her through it. And she said, 'I'm afraid I'm going to do something drastic.' I don't know if she meant to kill him or kill herself, but it didn't matter. We would never judge her.

"It has to be a group you're comfortable with," Jackie says, pointing a finger. "You need a good facilitator. I talk out at the meetings, and I'm very honest, which sometimes is shocking to people. This one woman's husband is in the beginning stages, but she told me, 'Don't ever stop coming. I've learned so much from you.'

"Thank God I got with the group," she says, shaking her head. "We all can laugh, and talk, and tell sad things. You cry, and when you walk out of there you think, 'Thank God I can do this for another week.' It was a tremendous help to me.

"Like I said, it's a bitch session for the caregivers," she says. "We all *know* what's coming, and our loved ones are in the other room singing *Joy to the World*."

She suddenly sits up straight. "Cosmo!" Jackie barks, "What are you chewing?"

The dog stares back at her.

She twists her lips, then looks back at me. "Biff couldn't talk the last couple of years, but the one thing he could do was cuss." She throws out her hands. "You know, like 'F, F, F, F, F.'" She says the letter, but not the word.

"All he could do was drop the F-bomb. He'd point at something he wanted, like this." She jabs a finger at the plate of cookies and says, "F, F, F, F, *F!*" stressing the final F.

"I would get frustrated, let me tell you. He'd sit there and I'd give him a cookie and say, 'Eat over the table,' and he'd sit back and put crumbs all over the floor. Yes, I would fuss at him. It's exasperating when these things happen. I'd put his oatmeal down, and next thing you know, his hands are in it. I'm like, 'Holy crap! What the hell?!' And he'd be like, 'F, F, F, F, *F!*'" And you almost had to laugh.

"One time, in Walmart, he walked away from me and I was horrified. I'm walking through the store yelling, 'Biff!' People were staring, but I didn't care. And there he was wandering through the store. I said, 'What were you doing?' and he said, 'Looking.'

"He could say words here or there, but one thing he always got out were those cuss words. He would have these little meltdowns and just fly off in these rages of frustration. He would cuss me out, but that was not his way. He thought I was the greatest thing since

Wheaties. After his temper tantrum he would just look at me and say, 'I love you.'"

She points at the pantry door behind her. "I kept this list on the wall of things you don't do: 'Don't argue with them. Don't debate things. Don't ask them their opinion.' Then I'd say, 'Why am I yelling at him?' It's not that he's doing this intentionally."

She takes a breath, then nods her head. "But I didn't feel guilty about that. I loved him dearly. I was very good to him. I took excellent care of him. I'd bathe him and get in the shower, and I'd say, 'Wash your hands, Biff,' and he'd wash his privates. I'd laugh and he'd laugh back, but he didn't know why he was laughing."

"Almost every Sunday we'd go to Cracker Barrel with friends. I had to feed him." She raises her chin and her eyes have that Jackie Campbell glint. "I was not ashamed of him. He couldn't help what he had. People stared and I got used to that. I didn't care.

"Biff's whole life revolved around me. He would follow me if I took the trash out. For the past two years, if I went to the bathroom, he stood at the door. He was afraid, and I was his security. As long as he had me, he felt okay. I took excellent care of him. Everybody kept saying, 'Jackie, you look terrible.' Buffy said, 'Mom, he's killing you. You have to put him in a home.' I thought, when Biff no longer knew who I was I'd have to put him away, but I couldn't do it to him. That would have ripped my heart out, because I knew how much he depended on me. I could see the fear in his eyes when I left his sight.

"I would shop when he was sleeping. I could leave him for short periods. He never left the house. Then, toward the end, my friend would come and sit with him. I took him every place with me up until the last. I took him to the grocery store, and he'd hold onto the cart.

"At home I bathed him, brushed his teeth, shaved him, and dressed him. He stood there like a mannequin. I had to feed him, or he would have eaten with his hands. I'd sit him in his green chair and turn on the TV, but he didn't know whether it was a football game or baseball. He'd wander around just touching things. He was like that from about three months ago. I think he was steadily going downhill the past six months."

I glance at the clock. We've been chatting for over an hour. I give Jackie a breather for a minute while I eat one of the cookies. It tastes as good as it looks.

"Do you like mincemeat?" she asks.

I wrinkle my nose and shake my head. "I never have."

"That's mincemeat in those cookies," she says, smiling, as if she's pulled one over on me, which she has.

I drink a sip of water and brace myself for the next part of the interview. I've heard bits and pieces of what Jackie went through only weeks earlier, and I know it won't be easy for her to relive it.

"Are you ready to talk about last month?"

Her smile straightens into a grim line, and she nods.

"It started December first. Biff had some blood work done, and I took him to the VA clinic to get the results. They have this luxury building over there, but they do not know how to deal with Alzheimer's patients.

"So we get there and the lady that takes you in to see the doctor weighed him and wanted to have him sit down. When people with Alzheimer's get to the end stages, they lose their depth perception. I'd have to move his chair around for him so he would feel secure to sit down. They don't see where the chair is."

Jackie stands and mimics guiding Biff into a chair.

"When the woman told him to sit down, he got antsy, so she grabbed his arm and shoulder and tried to guide him into the chair."

She places both hands on me and demonstrates. Her firm grip is startling.

"You don't force Alzheimer's patients to do anything," she says. "They stiffen. They're frightened. He grabbed her like a vice."

I ask how he grabbed the woman and Jackie clamps a hand over my forearm.

"She was about a hundred and fifty pounds, five-foot-four, and middle-aged. She got frightened and screamed for security."

Jackie is back in her chair now and she imitates the woman's cries: "Security! Security!"

"The more excited Biff got, the more frightened that girl got. He was babbling. He was nonverbal. It was mayhem. Two big black guys in security uniforms came. It took both of them just to get his hand off her forearm. Finally they got her out of the room."

Jackie takes a deep breath. "Then the police show up. Two of them, in uniform. Biff is sitting in the chair now because I said, 'Sit down, Biff, sit down.'

"Now these three women come in. Social workers. One said she'd worked with Alzheimer's patients and she knew you couldn't put your hands on them. Next thing you know, this man came in. He was the director of the VA clinic. All these people were in this little cubbyhole with us. I knew Biff was horrified.

"A crowd was gathering around the door, so I said, 'Excuse me. This is not a circus act!' They were gawking, and I said, 'Are you here to help my husband?'

"The police called me outside and asked questions. I said, 'Why are you here?' They said, 'We have to arrest your husband. He assaulted her.' I said, 'He did not assault her! He has stage three Alzheimer's. She grabbed him first!' They finally said they wouldn't charge him, but they wrote a report. Then the woman came back and apologized. She said, 'I'm sorry, Mrs. Campbell, but I never had to deal with that before.'"

Jackie takes a long sip of coffee before going on.

"So I got back in the room and I said to the director, 'I'm going to take him home,' and he said, 'No. You can't. You're going to have to invoke the Baker Act.'"

She explains that the Baker Act is a Florida law allowing for involuntary commitment for up to seventy-two hours of a person who has a mental illness and is deemed a harm to self or others.

"He said they were going to send him to a hospital in Ocala, and I said, 'Oh no, you're not! I'm going to take him home.'

"Meanwhile, the only thing you could understand my husband saying was cuss words. He's dropping the f-bomb all over the place.

He's saying, 'It's you! It's you! F-you, you bitch!' He was a racetracker. They would cuss all the time, but that reinforced their decision.

"They put me in another room separate from him. Next thing you know, police put handcuffs on him and took him away in a police car. They took him to Ocala and said I couldn't see him for seventy-two hours. I called and asked if I could come after the seventy-two hours. They said I could, but they only allowed visitors from six-thirty to seven at night in the psych ward, and I can't drive at night. They kept him for five days. Every time I called they said he was sleeping."

Her eyes are dry and steely as she recounts the nightmare.

"I don't know what happened to him in that hospital. They sent him to Arbor Village after that, and when he got there, he was black and blue up his arms and on his behind. They told me he fell out of bed. His nose was broken in two places. They said he fell on his face. I went back to the hospital and got the medical reports. They gave him like fifty milligrams of Seroquel, I don't know how many times a day. I went on the Internet and found that Seroquel and Alzheimer's don't mix."[2]

Jackie is becoming more agitated.

"When he got to Arbor Village he never regained consciousness. I went to visit him every day, and every time I went there he was like this." She closes her eyes, throws back her head, and makes loud raspy noises in her throat. "I was so afraid he was going to swallow his tongue. He was rigid. When you tried to lift his head, he was rigid.

"Monday night the girl called me and said they were taking him to the hospital. They didn't like how he was responding or breathing. They sent him to our local hospital, and he was there

2   According to Dr. Amanda G. Smith, M.D., Medical Director, USF Health Alzheimer's Center: Seroquel is an atypical antipsychotic. The FDA has a black box warning for this class of drugs, as it can increase the risk of stroke and death in the demented elderly. However, it can be an effective treatment for the delusions, hallucinations, and agitation seen in Alzheimer's disease when used appropriately and in low doses.

from Monday to Wednesday, but he never regained consciousness. I stayed with him night and day. He was like a vegetable. I said, 'Please God, take him.' His quality of life at home was zero.

"That whole thing has made me a firm believer in the power of prayer and that comatose people can hear you, because I called my daughter and said she had to come. She drove sixteen hours straight through, even though she had the flu. I begged him, 'Buffy's coming and she wants to see you.'

"His blood pressure was fifty-nine over twenty-seven. Can you imagine? I said, 'Come on, Biff, you've got to get out of this bed.' I actually poked him in the head to wake him up," Jackie says, poking herself in the forehead to demonstrate.

"I want to believe in my heart he knew Buffy was coming. He died twenty-five minutes after she got there. Buffy was sitting there holding his hand, and she said, 'Go on to Rhodes, Dad, he's waiting.'"

Jackie's face turns bright red, and for the first time she loses her composure. She speaks now through her sobs. "She was holding his hand, and she said, 'Mom I don't think he's breathing,' and he wasn't. It was quiet and it was peaceful. He just eased right on out."

Biff was seventy-two years old, one year older than Jackie. She looks across the room and says, "Biff always watched football on Sunday nights, and last night I looked at his green chair and I said, 'Yes, I miss you.'"

She can barely get the words out, but after a few deep breaths, she says, "It's lonely, but . . . that's the only thing I have to suffer now."

She wipes roughly at her face and apologizes for crying.

When I tell her she has nothing to apologize for, she insists, "I took excellent care of him. I'm glad God took him, because he had no quality of life, but when they took him away from me, that was awful. I don't want him to think I left him. It hurts me to think he'd think that. I had looked into Arbor Village. I said the first of the year that I might have to put him in there, because he'd fallen a couple of times, but I never had to make that decision."

Her eyes are dry again, and the glint is back. "I don't have any guilt about Biff. None at all. I prayed and prayed for God to do what was best for him. I think God was never going to take him unless He showed me it was time for him to go. By putting him through that ordeal, that's how He took him."

Jackie gets up from her chair and brings me a card given to her in memory of her husband. "He was a hard worker. He was a good provider, very personable. He never told me no. We had tragedy; we lost our son. That's the ultimate tragedy, but during that time I never thought of ever leaving Biff. I thought of murder a lot of times, but never divorce."

It is a relief to see her laugh.

She continues, "I don't regret or resent anything I did. I prayed constantly for God. I have a picture in the other room of Jesus. He's actually smiling in that picture. Did you ever see a picture with Jesus smiling? I would get on my knees in front of that picture and cry, and say, 'Give me guidance. I don't know what to do!' and He sent me the strength to take care of Biff. He gave me guidance: *'Here's what you have to do, Jackie.'* He was with me every day and walked with me. "

She sets her coffee mug down hard and says, "That's my story, and I'm sticking to it. When I lay my head on my pillow at night, my conscience is clear. I loved Biff. We had a great life. We had plans, and they didn't happen, but we had a fun life.

"I'll tell you what the real Alzheimer's is," she says. "It's *a living Hell* for the caregiver. It is a living Hell because you never know what to expect. You really don't know how to handle it emotionally. It can pull you down. I know it did me, and I really didn't think it would.

"A caregiver needs a support group. That is so important. I realize now how important that support group was to me. And you have to know yourself as the caregiver. Each caregiver has a different level—when you can't take it anymore—and you have to do something for your own sanity.

"You have to make yourself the priority, because your life is going to go on. As long as you know in your heart that you have done everything possible for that person, you have to take care of yourself. Don't be a martyr.

"When I lay the heavy stuff on people in the group in the beginning stages, they don't see it coming. We all have these safety valves that make us say, 'That's not going to happen to me.'"

She pauses and nods slowly. "I never saw myself wiping my husband's behind as I looked down the road to my future, but the love of a relationship makes you do what you have to do."

She sighs and looks out the window. "There's a man down the street whose wife has Alzheimer's, and I want to invite him to come to our group. The men who do come, it's very helpful to them. The man who now leads the respite care said he never went to a support group in the twelve years of his wife's Alzheimer's. He regrets that now, and says this is his way of giving back."

I turn off the tape recorder and thank Jackie for her time. Before I leave, I ask her to show me her favorite picture of Biff. She smiles and leads me to the living room. On the way she points and says, "That's the last birthday card he got." The card shows a caricature of a horse, laughing.

"This is Biff," she says, pointing to a photo on the wall of a smiling man with thinning hair and sparkling eyes. "And this is him not too long ago," she says, pointing to a photo inches away from the first. "See the difference?"

I do. The sparkle is gone.

She sniffs. "That's what the Alzheimer's did."

She points to another photo high up on the wall, and says, "That's my son."

Jackie was right. Rhodes was a big man . . . a strapping, handsome man in the prime of his life. He's standing arm in arm with a smiling woman in her twenties with long, dark hair and equally dark eyes.

"That was his fiancée," Jackie says. She explains that the photo was taken at the wedding of their best friend. "She and Rhodes were so close that the groom made both of them Best Man."

I laugh with her, and as I turn to leave she points to a large frame on the wall. "That's the picture of Jesus I told you about."

I stare in surprise. "That's some big smile."

She nods, and indicates an antique piece of furniture under the portrait. "A man came to refinish this old record cabinet a while back.

It was my mother's. He saw that painting of Jesus, and he commented on it, because you never see pictures of Him smiling like that."

Jackie tilts her head and gazes at the portrait. She is smiling too, now, even after recounting the long ordeal that she's been through.

"I think that man was offended by the picture," she says, "but I like it."

She glances at Biff's empty chair, then looks back at the smiling Jesus. Her voice is wistful as she concludes, "It makes me feel good."

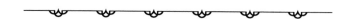

Judy smiles at a large woman with thick hair the color of straw. "Okay, Mary?"

One smile from Mary and the group perks up. "I had a wonderful Christmas. My two sons came down, and they stayed at a hotel, so it wasn't all crazy."

"That's a good idea," Judy tells the group. "Sometimes too much activity in the house can make a person with Alzheimer's more agitated."

Mary nods. "Yes, but then on Tuesday night after Christmas, everybody was gone and my mom was sitting there crying. She said, 'I just can't believe it's Christmas, and my grandchildren didn't call me.' She had totally forgotten that they were here, and she was so sad. It broke my heart to see her like that. I said, 'Mom, that was four days ago! You don't remember?' and she didn't remember.

"So I hugged her, and she went to bed, but it startled me. She'd been doing so well, and then not to remember such a special day . . . . It just really hurt."

The others listen attentively. There is no judgment, only understanding.

"So, you just don't know what to expect," Mary concludes. "I mean, the best day can turn into the worst day. But she's okay now. She remembers again, so that was just a blip."

7

FAMILY HISTORY

"WHEN THE NEUROLOGIST TOLD ME my mother was in the early stages of Alzheimer's," says Carol Haimbaugh, an attractive woman of sixty-eight with short blond hair and thin features, "I was like, '*Oh, shit*.' I didn't know much about it at the time, but I knew it was something I didn't want in my family.

"They asked about my family's medical history, and I told them my father had been diagnosed with Alzheimer's. The doctor looked at me and said, 'You have both parents with Alzheimer's. That puts you in the ninety-five percent category. You need to pay attention to yourself.' That threw me into a state of high anxiety, so that's when I started my journey of researching and learning. I was worried about her, but I was also worried about me."

Carol sits with her husband Dick at a wooden table in a kitchen that overlooks a built-in pool and a golf course beyond. Dick, dressed in a burgundy polo shirt and golf shorts, is seventy-five, but he looks no older than his wife. The atmosphere in their designer home is informal and relaxed, which is how the two of them come across as they share their story.

Carol speaks proudly of her mother. "She's spry, pretty, and a very young ninety. She worked as a shampoo girl, standing on her feet until she was eighty-one, which is the same age she was diagnosed with Alzheimer's."

Dick says, "She had elements of the disease that we didn't recognize before the diagnosis."

Carol nods in agreement. "She lived and worked in Chicago, and I started getting calls. Her two girlfriends told me, 'There's something not right with your mother.' I would visit her and see no evidence. About a year later, she did say, 'I'm having trouble with my checkbook,' or 'Sometimes I get a little confused, and I'm worried I might not pay my taxes.' So those were the first clues.

"I sat down with her one day, and I found her checkbook to be a mess, which was not how I knew my mom to be. She was very independent. She'd been on her own for ten years, and we never worried at all about her. We weren't thinking Alzheimer's; we were thinking normal aging.

"We talked with her doctor, and he confirmed the concept that we all start to slip a little around age eighty. He did the typical Alzheimer's test." Carol holds out her hand and says, "You know, the 'remember five items' thing. They tell you five items, and you have to remember them."

"She's always been very good when interviewed by a doctor," Dick says.

"And she did great on that test," Carol confirms, "so we continued for two years, just following up. From what we know today, I think further testing would have helped, but back then more testing wasn't considered.

"She finally quit working, because it was hard on her back. Then things started to show up more. She had more time on her hands. She wasn't interacting with people all day, and she wasn't challenged."

"She was becoming more reclusive," Dick says. "She started to withdraw."

Carol says, "Years later she told me that she started withdrawing when she realized she couldn't remember people's names and other details that she should recall. That frightened her. She was afraid to be put in a position where people would notice. So it was a conscious decision at that point, but it was changing her quality of life.

"We made a decision to put her in an independent living facility near her friends. She could get her meals there. She chose the building, and she was very happy about it initially. Everything looked like it was going to work out real well. The problem is, you take them out of a familiar environment, and there's an emotional effect. We didn't realize it would make her so confused."

Dick nods in agreement as Carol continues.

"She wanted to know why she wasn't home. She would be confused about why she wasn't in her own place, and then her confusion would clear up. That still happens today. Every day she asks me, 'Why am I living here?' She has told us over the years of her Alzheimer's, 'I'm fine. I'm okay. I'll tell you when it's time to come live with you.' But that time came faster than she thought, so we brought her to live with us."

Dick says, "She was in independent living for two years, then she lived with us for five years in Illinois and in Florida, and then we moved her into the home she's in now."

"She's back in independent living now," Carol clarifies, "with services. She was here in Florida with us, and she turned a corner mentally. She went through a period of being suspicious and fearful.

"She had little things happen, like one day when she thought her rings were missing. It became an obsession, so I went out and bought her fake rings—just costume jewelry—and she went, 'Oh, God, I have my rings!' And she was happy again.

"Oh, that's one thing—" Carol adds, "When someone with Alzheimer's says something that you know is inaccurate, don't correct them. They don't understand. You need to just agree with them and give them some assurance that they're thinking okay."

Dick jumps in, "Or distract them. I have one thing that always works with her mother. Always."

Carol laughs and glances at the ceiling. She knows what he's going to say.

"Fifteen years ago," Dick says, "we were at a casino, and Carol's mother borrowed a hundred dollars from me. She paid it back, but now, any time she needs distraction, I'll say to her, 'What about that hundred dollars you owe me?' And right away she'll say, 'I paid you that hundred dollars!' It jerks her right out of whatever she was thinking about."

"We have a lot of fun with that," Carol confirms. "It's a great distraction." She pauses and takes a deep breath. The energy in the kitchen shifts as she begins to describe a pivotal incident that no one found humorous.

"About two years ago I was putting some clean clothes away in my mother's room, and she noticed me closing a drawer. She came out of her room shortly thereafter and said, 'Why did you take my money?' I said, 'I didn't take any money. You don't have any money in your drawer.' But she accused me of stealing from her, and that really hurt."

Dick says, "That's when she decided she wanted to move out."

"That really hurt," Carol repeats. "On one level, you know it's the illness talking, but on another level, it's the real person talking. You know logically that you're talking to a damaged brain, but all you hear is your mother accusing you of stealing from her and abandoning her. No matter how well you know what's going on, you still hurt."

Dick gives his wife a sympathetic look, and says, "When that happens, there's no way I can give Carol enough support to help her."

"He'll put his arm around me," Carol says, "but there's nothing he can say to make the hurt go away. She doesn't even live with us anymore, and it still hurts every day." She glances at the telephone. "She's already called two times today. The responsibility doesn't go away just because she's not living with us."

Carol describes the unexpected changes that came about when she started caring for her mother.

"When we first brought her to live with us, I began to give up my life, but I didn't' recognize it. I had retired from the work world and had a working art studio in my house in Illinois. It was great fun." She throws her head back. "Oh, my God, it was so much fun. I was having the time of my life, and it ended," she says, slapping her hand on the table, "just like that.

"The wall came down overnight. Her needs just absorbed our life, even though she wasn't a needy person. Whatever she needed, we had to do: take her to the doctor, take her to get her hair done—do all these things for another person who can't do them. Your life is completely changed, because there's no time for yourself.

"I didn't recognize how much I was giving up, how much I was no longer *me*. I was losing myself in the process."

"And she was in denial that this was happening," Dick says. "I saw the effect on her—things like her concern that we couldn't go away, because Carol would say, 'Who's going to stay with Mom?' So it brought our life in," he brings his hands close together, "but she was in total denial, because of her concern and love for her mother."

"Dick was never angry," Carol says. "He was never jealous." She puts her hand on his arm. "He was always loving and interactive with her, but he would comment that I needed to do more for myself. He was being my caregiver, while I was being the caregiver to my mother."

Dick gives a modest shrug.

"I hadn't realized I needed my artwork so much," Carol goes on. "It was keeping me grounded. That was my form of refilling my spiritual fuel, and when I cut off my connection to it, I started getting more and more diminished. I started getting more and more depressed.

"So I kept deteriorating, but I didn't recognize it. When you're caught in that state, you can't make the decision to get out of it. I went to doctors who said, 'Oh, we'd better put you on some anti-depressive medication.' I tried two different medicines, but they just put me in a bit of a stupor. So, I didn't have anxiety attacks, but I wasn't functioning. I wasn't happy. I didn't recognize that it was part of this 'caregiver's syndrome.'"

Dick says, "She masked it very well when her mother was with us, up to the point where they had the episode with the accusations."

Carol purses her lips. "The year prior to that was when things were really difficult for me. From a spiritual level, I knew that I was not supposed to be taking care of my mother anymore. I knew my life was not good. I had financial security, a wonderful husband, gifts and talents, and none of the depression was due to these things. My life was simply out of balance from taking care of my mother.

"I remember thinking, 'What is wrong?' and I saw a wheel in my mind, but it couldn't move because it was flat. I'm thinking, 'What the hell is this flat wheel?' It looked like a pie, and this huge piece of the pie looked like it was flat. That piece was caring for my mother. That was part of my, 'Oh, my God.' But did I say, 'I need to make a change here?' No. I had to take care of her, because I had a very close bond with my mom, and I remember promising her when I was a little girl that I would take care of her forever.

"So I was literally losing my life, trying to take care of my mother. It's so easy to fall prey to the self deception that we are handling the stress of the change in our lives just fine, but I started recognizing that I really shouldn't be doing this. I really needed to find another opportunity for her. This was not the way I wanted my life to go, but I wasn't making any changes. I kept going, constantly ruminating. That was my Higher Self trying to get my attention. I got so many messages that I ignored, then I got a spiritual 2x4 between the eyes."

Dick realizes that Carol hasn't explained what the 2x4 was, so he announces, "She had a stroke in the car while driving her mother to get her hearing aid fixed."

Carol explains, "We were in Illinois. Dick was driving, and Mom was in the back seat. I was reading the street signs, and all of a sudden I saw the letters fall off a sign. They just fell off, and the sign was blank. I thought, 'Oh, that's weird.'"

She puts her hand flat against her chest as she says, "Then I had this feeling like you have when you're going down a roller coaster, and I said to Dick, 'I think there's something wrong.'

"A FedEx truck pulled in front of us, and I saw those big letters on the side fall off. Then I punched Dick in the arm and said, 'There's something wrong! The letters are falling off!' I got a map out and I was looking at blank paper. There were no letters. Dick pulled over, and I called my doctor on my cell phone."

Dick jumps in, "She described to the doctor what was happening, and the doctor said, "Go to the hospital. There must be some-thing disruptive happening in your brain.'"

"We were three blocks from the hospital," Carol says, "when all the letters came back, so I talked him into taking me to Mom's appointment. That's how stubborn caregivers are.

"We went to the hearing appointment and got that taken care of, and we started on our way back home. Dick asked me, 'Do you want to go to the hospital now?' and when I went to answer, the words came out, '*Blah, blah, blah.*'"

She says this in a goofy voice while making a comical face.

"We went straight to the hospital," Carol says. "I went up to the triage desk and went, '*Blah, blah, blah,*' and they took me right in. They did all the tests, and a neurologist said my films looked very suspicious.

"I was there for two days, and then—this was foolish—I said, 'Let's go back to Florida. I'll get a neurologist there.' So we came back with Mom. I should have stayed in Illinois and gone to the neurologist that I knew there. What happened is, I came back here, and the symptoms began to show up. I didn't look any different, but problems started to occur. We ended up going back to Illinois, to a stroke specialist."

Dick says, "The doctor asked, 'Is anything different in your life to have precipitated this?' and Carol said, 'Well, my mother's living with us.' And *Bingo!*" he throws his hands out.

"During that time my sister said, 'I'm taking Mom.' She's twelve years younger than I am and works full time. She still had a teenager in high school. We knew her lifestyle was going to change dramatically, so we took the summer to find a place where Mom could live. We put her in the independent living home where she lives now. My sister takes Mom to her house every weekend."

Carol explains that her mother's dementia hasn't progressed as quickly as most. "She is ninety years old, and she is bright, and articulate . . . ."

Dick chimes in, "If her mother is out socially, she has learned to call everyone 'Honey.' You would have no idea she has Alzheimer's."

"Her neurologist is amazed at her," Carol says. "And I asked, 'Doesn't that strike you as odd after eight years that she's still able to live on her own?' and he said, 'It does strike me as odd.'

"It turns out that when she was twenty-five, she suffered a severe head concussion from her husband hitting her," Carol confides. "They didn't go to doctors about abuse in those years, but when she finally did, it was too late. Her eardrum was shattered. The doctor concluded the likelihood is that she got Alzheimer's from head trauma, and her medication helped delay things.

"Still," Carol admits, "There are days she doesn't remember talking to me, so she does have severe memory loss.

"If I call after four o-clock in the afternoon, that's when she's starting to sundown. She'll say, 'I need to ask you, why am I here? I thought I was supposed to be with you.'

The reason her mother is no longer living with her, Carol explains, is that after her stroke, Carol needed to focus on retraining her brain.

"The incident with the accusations happened in February two years ago, and the stroke was in April. She went into the home in August, and we came back here without her in September. I started my rehab immediately to get back up to speed."

Carol could tell she wasn't completely normal. "I used to design art and sewing patterns for classes that I gave. I would write out all the instructions. I decided I wanted to make some patterns for one of my nephews, and I couldn't remember how to do it. I had forgotten."

When asked if the forgetfulness could be an early sign of Alzheimer's, Carol admits that she doesn't know for sure.

"Honestly," she says, "I haven't set that out as a possibility. I think mine is from the stroke damage. I could not follow the instructions, so somewhere there's a disconnect. I called the neurologist and asked, 'Could this be from the stroke?' and he said, 'Yes, it could.'

In spite of being so far from her mother now, Carol and Dick remain quite involved in her life.

"We still take care of all of her legal and financial issues, and I still interface with her physician on the phone. I talk to my sister probably three times a week. I call my mother every day to remind her to do things.

"We leave Florida for about four months each year and return to northern Illinois to take over for my sister. That gives her a few months of normalcy. When we're up there, Mother spends every Sunday at our house, plus we take her for an outing every week. Then we do another half-day visit with her at her apartment to play cards and watch TV, or maybe do a little laundry, or visit a local Walgreens for shopping." She notes that Alzheimer's patients easily get overwhelmed in big stores, but that smaller drugstores have a bit of everything.

"I take her to her doctor's appointments, manicure appointments, and to visit her friends. These are things my sister does during the year, and things that I did when she lived with me, but now we have the relief of taking her back to her apartment, and having space to become ourselves again. Loss of identity is a terrible consequence of this lifestyle, and is what led to my anxiety, depression and eventual stroke.

"Handling the full burden of another person's financial and legal issues is still very difficult," Carol says. "Each year I'm responsible for refiling for her supplemental and drug insurances, and the rules change every year, so it takes investigation. We also have to resubmit all the required information to the Veteran's Assist program. These are all complicated, and I dread them every year. I can't imagine what people who aren't aware about the changes do about these types of things.

"So, you see, even when you have the blessing of having them living somewhere else, you continue to dedicate a good deal of your time to their life." She shakes her head. "There's an army of us out there doing all this, pretty much alone. That incident where she accused me of taking her money triggered the stress. Here I thought I was doing so much for her . . . ."

"She was," Dick insists.

"I was fortunate that my stroke debilitations were such that a year of rehab and continuing attention were able to restore me to minor physical and mental challenges that I can work around," Carol says. "Not every caregiver is as lucky. People should seriously consider that if they become debilitated, the person they are sacrificing themselves for will no longer have the loving care they were trying to give.

"Placing them in an appropriate facility with active involvement is a much better solution. Financial help is sometimes more available than people know." She chops a hand through the air and insists, "They are not abandoning their loved one. They are making sure they'll be around to love them for a much longer time."

She now deals with her stress in a more positive way than in the past.

"I've added a spiritual component to caring for myself," Carol says, "During that time when I was feeling bad about not having her live with me anymore, I received some good advice. It was simply to send her love. I got inspired to create a meditative program just for dealing with my mother."

She sits back and her face takes on a dreamy look as she describes her meditation.

"I open my heart to her and hold an image of her being very happy. I see her eyes twinkling, and she is smiling, as if she's enjoying the company of family members she loves. In the background are a couple of large angels making sure she feels their affection and presence, so that no matter any confusion in her state of mind, she knows that she is loved and not alone. Sometimes I just imagine she is being held and comforted.

"I usually cry once I've gotten a picture in place, but it's cathartic. I finish up with a deep breath or two, and I feel a bit better because I am doing *something* by sending this love.

"I also continue to go to the support group that I've been going to on and off for eight years," she says. "I started going as soon as Mom was diagnosed. When we moved here I went to a group called, 'Parents in the Home.' It wasn't restricted to people with

Alzheimer's, but now I go to a group here just for people with Al-zheimer's. It puts things in perspective. You start to ask questions, and you begin to get a picture of what kind of resources and services are available to you. They talk about things you don't know unless you go to these meetings."

Dick says, "There are a lot of doctors who aren't very good at treating Alzheimer's patients. So, by going to those meetings you hear who's really good."

"The groups can't endorse someone," Carol adds, "but the people at the meetings are a good source of referrals.

"Most importantly, there's compassion that gets shared at those meetings, and even if you say nothing, you're absorbing that compassion. There's an unstated love that's transferred around the group. Nobody has to say it. It's just that realization that there's another person who's hurting like you're hurting."

Carol turns to Dick, and they share a knowing look. There is an unstated love between them as well.

Dick takes a deep breath, then says, "We're doing the best we can for ourselves and the very best we can for her mom. We make sure that she is well taken care of and that she knows she is loved."

"Initially," Carol says, "I was so scared because of the stroke that I was relieved my mother was no longer living with us. I was grateful that I could work on me, and redirect all the energy I'd been pouring out on her. I knew she was safe and well taken care of. My sister doesn't get sucked in like I do. She doesn't carry the guilt thing. I'm a little too sensitive.

"Because of my family history, my physician did do the blood test to see whether I have the Alzheimer's factor in my blood." She nods toward a credenza by the front door. "The report is sitting in the desk over there, and it says, yes, I do have the factor."

A pregnant pause follows, then Carol fills in the silence.

"We don't know where I am as far as my condition. I did get a baseline done, but I haven't gone back for any more follow-ups, because I don't want to see where I am."

Dick makes a face and gives a dismissive shake of his head.

"You don't need to go back for a follow-up. I can testify to that."

Carol gives him an appreciative smile, then sums up her attitude.

"I don't live my life with fears."

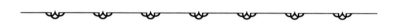

A woman on the far side of the room raises her hand. "Is it okay to ask a question?"

"Of course," says Judy. "That's one of the reasons we come here—to get answers."

"Well," the woman says, my husband can't tell time anymore. Every five minutes he's asking me the same thing."

"May I suggest something?" says a lady five seats to the left. "It's the hands on the clock that confuse them, so I bought my husband a digital clock."

"We have one," the woman replies, "He wanted a digital watch, but now I have to figure out how to set the time."

Judy says, "That's very normal, let me tell you. I shopped for weeks to find a watch that had nothing on it except the clock . . . none of those gadgets and buttons. Chuck would play with all the gadgets, and I didn't know how to fix them." She crosses her hands back and forth. "No, no, no. Definitely no gadgets. Go out and get the plain watch. It's out there.

"Connie?" Judy nods at the next woman.

"Our Christmas was a complete bust," Connie says. "He woke up in the morning and said, 'I don't feel good,' and he went back to bed. That was so unusual, because he's pretty social. He loves to sing karaoke. So I emailed Judy and said, 'What do I do?' She said, 'Forget it. It's okay.'"

Others listen with concern as Connie tells about the rest of her holiday. "So he slept the whole day. All day long. I did wake him up for dinner, and he's been fine since, but I had no idea what was going on. We were invited to quite a large party with all our golfing friends, but he just didn't want to go. So, we had pizza for Christmas, and that was it." She shrugs and adds an incongruous, "And that was fine."

All present know that it wasn't really fine, but Judy sums it up.

"You got through it."

She turns to the next woman. "Okay, tell them life goes on."

8

THE VOICE OF REASON

WHEN JACKIE PRESTON PUT HER HUSBAND HOMER in a nursing home, the staff came running. They thought a famous TV starlet had arrived. The staff was disappointed. It turns out that Jackie wasn't Rue McClanahan from *The Golden Girls*, but they could be forgiven for thinking she was. Even Jackie can see the resemblance.

Jackie is a young seventy-five. She projects warmth and carries herself with quiet self-assuredness—the perfect attributes for her volunteer work as an Alzheimer's support group facilitator. Her other qualification for the job is the time she spent caring for Homer, who passed away five years earlier at age 79.

"He was diagnosed nine years ago," Jackie tells me as we sit on a couch in her cozy living room. "The reason I know for a fact when it was, is that's the year I was diagnosed with lung cancer. I already suspected there was something wrong with Homer before then. He knew something was going on, too. I'd only known him a few years at the time, and he was sort of an eccentric person anyhow. Had I known him longer, I might have recognized it sooner."

Jackie seems completely at ease discussing her husband's illness. "He went for testing, and they kept him all day. They did all the memory tests, of course, but no medical tests. They said he was fine, which I knew was not the truth. I had worked with the elderly for many years as a manager of housing for low income seniors. I was aware of Alzheimer's, only in that some of my people in the buildings had it, but I was not really that familiar with the disease.

"After he got the diagnosis that he was fine, I was diagnosed with the lung cancer, so concerns about his memory sort of fell by the wayside. I went through surgery and had my upper right lobe removed. Thank God, they got it all, but while I was going through the surgery, Homer became totally disoriented.

"See, it was the trauma of having all this happen to me," Jackie explains. "He just went off the deep end. The day he came to the hospital to pick me up, I'd been in there for a week and had just had the drains taken out of my chest. I was incapacitated and unable to do anything. Homer didn't know where he was, why he was there, or where he had parked. He got to my room, and he just sort of fell apart. They didn't even want him to take me home. I said 'No, no!' I could guide him home if they could find the car.

"As soon as I was able, I made an appointment with a neurologist. They put him through all the testing, with a PET scan and everything. It was Alzheimer's. He was put on medications, and there wasn't much I could do at that point, because I was bedridden for a while."

A ginger-colored cat steps into the room, and seeing that there is a guest in the house, she stops. I ask what the cat's name is, and learn that she is appropriately named Ginger. She looks as if she wants to come closer, but then decides to leave.

Jackie continues, "Homer was in and out. He didn't stay in that confused state all the time. He came back a little bit. I realized then that this is how the disease works. You don't get back what you had before. It's lost. It's gone. It may come back in little dribs and drabs, but certain things just go.

"Around that time, we visited his cousin in Leesburg, Florida, and she asked if I'd ever seen The Villages. I said, 'Let's go look at it.' All I had to do was see all the golf courses, and I knew it was perfect. Homer was an avid golfer. His priority was always golf, me, and the children." She counts each priority off on her fingers, then adds, "and we all knew what came first." The tilt of her head shows that golf got top billing.

"He had lost his interest in golfing, so I said, 'Let's move there.' I thought it would renew his interest, but I was totally ignorant of the disease and how it worked. I was fooling myself. I realize now he was incapable of doing anything.

"Looking back," she says, "there were signs. Taking care of his money was always a big interest, then all of a sudden he turned over all of his finances to a financial advisor—an outsider. I should have known then that he knew something was going on.

"Another time before we even moved here, his grandson brought his girlfriend to visit. We had a perfectly lovely time, but after they left, Homer said, 'Explain to me who he is.' I said, 'Why, that's your grandson!' It was at that point that I knew. Every point I would know, and then things seemed to be straightened out a while, then the next thing would happen."

She runs her fingers through her short, blond hair. "I guess, in a way, you don't want to know. It's very difficult. But still, the ramifications weren't clear to me until I started researching it and realized that once these faculties are gone, they don't come back. But he enjoyed that young man's visit that day, and to think that all that time, he had no idea who he was! To me, that was unfathomable. That's when I realized that Alzheimer's patients are not living in the 'now,' they're living in the 'then.'"

Jackie clears her throat and excuses herself to get a cough drop. Ginger the Cat reappears, then does her vanishing act again. Jackie returns to the couch and picks up where she left off.

"Homer was still taking care of himself, if I told him to. I would set things up for him to shower and brush his teeth. One day he'd been in the bathroom a long, long time, so I walked in, and he was trying to brush his teeth with his razor." She shudders. "Luckily, I got there before he hurt himself. I said, 'No, no, no, Homer, that's not your toothbrush!' Of course I went out that day and bought a cordless electric razor."

She stares out the window for a moment, lost in the memory. "That was very scary," she admits.

"He would go into his bedroom and take all the underwear out of his drawers. He would put on undershorts, then maybe a pair of shorts and a golf shirt, then he would put on maybe two or three more pair of undershorts, then a sock on one foot, but no sock on the other foot. There was no way I could convince him that he had too many clothes on. It was a struggle. Eventually, I learned to just put in the drawer what he needed.

"He got in the habit of getting up in the middle of the night, getting himself all dressed, then waking me up to say, 'Come on. It's time to go.' I'd say, 'Go where?' and he'd say, 'Go home.' I'd tell him, 'We *are* home,' and he'd say, 'No, no, no, my mama needs me. We haven't seen her in a long time.' His mother was gone," Jackie explains, "but I learned to say, 'Homer, you know, your mama is in bed, and she's asleep. Let's wait until the morning, and when we get up we'll give her a call.' That would work," she says, "but it got to the point where I didn't do a whole lot of sleeping.

"Homer went to a facility for the last fourteen months of his life. His daily care and the responsibility became way more than I could handle. If he didn't want to do something, he didn't do it. He was never mean or nasty, as some of them get, but he was very firm about certain things. He never hurt me." She rolls her eyes, then adds, ". . . *intentionally.*" Jackie elaborates, "If I was trying to do something to keep him out of harm's way, he would take me by the arm to move me, and my arms were always bruised.

"Putting him in the home was one of the hardest things I ever had to do in my whole life. The only thing harder was losing a son to the AIDS virus just before I met Homer. The guilt of placing your loved one is terrible. You feel like you're throwing them away, and that you're not going to be the caregiver anymore. Ask anybody who has had to do it or has contemplated it. Most people keep them at home because they promise they will never put them in a home." She points a finger. "Do not ever promise that you won't place them. We tell people that all the time, because the guilt's bad enough even if you haven't promised them.

"I took a lot of time to find what I thought was the right home for him. His oldest son's wife came down and helped me make the decision. I took Homer over there a few times and we'd sit in the living room area for a few minutes so it wasn't totally unfamiliar to him. My youngest son was living nearby at the time, and if it hadn't been for him, it would have been a lot harder for me. He was there to talk to Homer and help get him settled in.

"When we started to leave he tried to follow us. They suggested that I not come back for a couple of days, which was hard. When I went back, he didn't seem to realize I'd been gone very long, if at all, but he thought that I'd come to get him and take him back. I would just go outside and cry. That's all you can do. You think, 'Can I take him back home and take care of him?' And of course, the answer is no.

"I finally hit on the solution to leaving. Homer had a very strong work ethic. When I would leave, he would say, 'Oh, do you have to go?' and I'd say, 'I have to go to work now, and I don't want to be late,' Jackie says, demonstrating the benefits of telling what Judy Simms calls a "fiblet."

"That worked for him. I even went away for two weeks on a cruise to Alaska with a friend. I had already planned this before he went in the home. A friend was going to stay with him, then we had to place him. The administrator said, 'Absolutely, go ahead with your plans. He will not know that you're not here every day.' So I went and I had a swell time, and when I came back, he had no recollection that I hadn't been there.

"It got to the point where Homer forgot my name, and he didn't understand 'wife' or relationships at all. He just knew I was someone he could trust. The only people he remembered were his mama and his brother when he was young."

Life settled into a routine for Jackie.

"I went to see him about every two or three days. After a while it wasn't so hard that he didn't know me, because my understanding of this disease showed me that it is what it is, and you can't change that. You have to accept it. Not everybody did, but that acceptance gave me a level of peace. I knew what the outcome would be."

She is very calm as she explains, "It's like a movie you're watching for the second time. You know what the ending is. I knew he was not going to live through this disease. I didn't know how long it would take, but the ending is always the same.

"After he got adjusted to the memory care unit, he was friendly with people. He was born in Alabama, and he was basically a southern gentleman. When dinnertime would come, he would go and find the smallest, most frail lady, and help her into the room. He got himself these little jobs to do. So I went in there to visit him one day with a neighbor. We walked in and he was standing there buttoning his shirt, and this woman walked out of his bathroom with her purse over her arm and I said, 'Oh, hello!'" Jackie raises her eyes just as she did at the time. "The woman said, 'My husband and I are getting ready to go out,' and I said to Homer, "Okay. Where are you going?' and he said, 'I don't know.'

"The woman just sat down with her purse, so I went to the nurses and explained what was going on. They got upset over it for me, but I told them I wasn't upset. They went and reminded her that he was not her husband. So I went back one day, and there in the living room is Homer sitting on the sofa. He has his arm around this same woman's shoulder, and she has her head on his shoulder. It was actually very sweet," Jackie says with sincerity.

"Homer motioned me over and put his arm around my shoulder. So there we were, the three of us, and the staff got all upset, but I said, "It's okay. If they get a little comfort, it's all right. As long as you can assure me you're not going to let them do anything improper, it's okay.' The other woman never said a word, but she never took her eyes off me." Jackie demonstrates how the woman glared, and says, "If looks could kill, I'd be dead!" Then she adds, "But I felt good about that, because it must have been some comfort for him.

"When I have told that story sometimes in our groups—" she pauses and mimics the startled faces, "—somebody would say, 'I would never let that happen! That just couldn't work!'" Jackie shrugs. "Jealousy has never been one of my problems in life.

"He lost his ability to verbalize very early on. By the time we put him in the home, he was not able to hold a conversation." She explains that as time passed, "He would jabber on and on, making no sense whatsoever. The words meant nothing, but he knew what he was saying. He knew, because he would stop talking and leave me room to make some kind of comment. When that first starts, you try to help them to get the right words out, but pretty soon it becomes apparent there's no point to it. As long as he was happy that I still responded, it was okay.

"At the end he just went way down. We were walking through the hallway one day, and he was jibber-jabbering to me. He had his arm through mine, and he stopped and said, clear as day, 'You'll never know how much I love you.' That was the last thing he said that made any sense. I was astonished. You want to say to yourself, 'Oh, he's getting better. This was all a dream.' And then he just drifted back to the way he was.

"Homer ultimately passed from the disease. Often, people with Alzheimer's who have other physical problems will die from a heart attack, but he died from the disease. It robs the brain of the ability to tell the body what to do. The brain controls everything, and it becomes so entangled that it stops telling you that you need to eat to stay alive. The brain doesn't say 'chew and swallow,' and eventually it doesn't tell you to take another breath."

Jackie describes his final days. "He stopped eating. I would go to feed him, and he had no clue what to do with the utensils. It got to the point where I would put the food in his mouth, and he would chew and swallow, then he would sit and look at me if I put it in his mouth. Then, after a while, it just fell right out. He had a 'Do Not Resuscitate' order and 'no heroic measures.' We had both decided those things long before anybody was sick.

"Hospice came in with him the last two weeks. He had an IV for hydration, but that's the only thing they did at the end. That's the way it goes for people who don't want to be hooked up to anything.

"The few years my husband and I had were very good years, with the exception of those last years that were so sad." She gives a wistful smile. "He was a real 'keeper,' and I'm so appreciative of the time we had together. We were good companions, good lovers, good everything, and I feel blessed to have known him."

She gazes out the window toward the golf course, then says, "I was more than happy to take care of him as well as I could, but very sorry that I had to.

"To me, the real Alzheimer's is the terrible loss of dignity and humanity. I don't think the patient has any concept of what Alzheimer's is, because they lose everything. They're like a shell. To me that's just the worst thing. They've lost their memories of their children, their livelihood, and their talents. The one bright spot is the fact that the person with the disease doesn't realize they have the disease. If they knew, it would be awful.

"Don't be afraid to talk to your neighbors and friends and tell them what your situation is. This is a very isolating disease, because others don't know what to say to the person with the Alzheimer's and to the person who's caring for them. They don't know how to offer to get involved, and they're afraid, 'What if this person gets violent, or tries to get away?' It's vital that the caregiver inform their neighbors.

"We have little cards that say, 'My companion has Alzheimer's. Please be patient.' You can show that to a server in a restaurant or in a grocery store, because the behavior is often bizarre. That's why I think you should let people know, so that if there is bizarre behavior, they don't go running down the street. It's not something you want to keep a secret.

"As a caregiver, don't let this take over your whole life. Try to do as many of the things you did before that you can still do. Try to find people that you can have come in and stay, even if you have to pay for it. Do anything you can to keep yourself a whole person. But most of all, get into a support group and be with people who understand what you're talking about and can give you some help with it."

Jackie is very matter-of-fact about what she went through, and she explains that this trait is part of her personality.

"I started being a group facilitator while my husband was still alive. They asked me to help facilitate because I had a bit more control over myself than the others because of my situation. I'll never forget their very words to me that day: 'Jackie, you're the only one in here that still has some sparkle in your eyes.'

"At the time I was more rational than a lot of people, just because of the way I am. I'm a Libra, and if we can't rationalize things, we'll go crazy. We have to make it right within ourselves. But," she pauses now to make a point, "I also was not married to that man for fifty years. That makes a big, big difference. Some of the caretakers have known no other life, and I think that makes all the difference in the world.

"I realize that when I'm working with caretakers as a facilitator, that they're not like me. So I tell them why it was different for me. They can be upset." She puts her hands out and says, "I don't know how you could help not be, but I also tell them it is what it is, and you have to realize that. You have to realize that it is not going to get better. A lot of people come to the support group meetings with the attitude that, 'We're here for you to help us make it better,' but there is no cure at this point for this disease.

"Sometimes the director of the Alzheimer's Family Organization will call me to say, 'I need to talk to the voice of reason.'" She makes a sheepish face. "I didn't know that's what I was, but I seem to be able to say the right thing and help people get settled down. I'm pretty logical."

Jackie Preston laughs, then shows that she doesn't take herself too seriously. "I can say things with great authority, and realize later on that I really don't know what I'm talking about. That's why my motto is 'Often wrong, but never in doubt!'"

She ends with a final piece of advice for caregivers. "Don't do this by yourself. Find a group so you can be with people who understand what you're talking about. The people around you who've never dealt with this don't and can't understand, and hopefully will never have to."

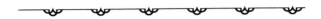

"I'm very happy," says the next woman, who looks anything but happy. Her face is drawn and lined, and gravity tugs firmly at the corners of her mouth.

"My husband passed in July. He was diagnosed with dementia. I still wrack my brain figuring out when it started, but you can't tell. You really can't."

"But now you're enjoying life again," Judy asserts.

"Yes," she says, and somehow, beneath her apparent lack of emotion, the words ring true.

Judy gives a firm nod. "Okay." She glances at the clock, then moves on to the next woman. "Veronica?"

Veronica gets straight to the point. "I got him not to drive, but I did it by lying. You really can't talk to him, but it took a little while for me to stretch the truth. Judy talked enough about telling "fiblets" that I said, 'You know, what's it gonna hurt if I just tell him a story?' And it worked. First time I tried it, and I thought, 'Gee, where've I been?' So it's just these little things you learn the hard way."

"And she's going to get all her paperwork in order," Judy says in a tone of voice not unlike a mother talking to a child. "So that's going to eliminate a lot of stress. We always encourage you to do that early—the wills and things."

It is a lesson, she tells the group, that some people only learn the hard way . . . .

9

A LACK OF TRUST

"MY HUSBAND'S NAME WAS RICHARD BAXTER, and he died two months ago. He was eighty-one. It was my second time to lose a husband. My first husband died of throat cancer."

Mary Baxter relates this information with no outward show of emotion. She comes across poised and proper. Her appearance is as stately as the large luxury home in which we meet. Her full, yellow-blond hair and perfectly manicured nails give the impression that she is no stranger to a beauty salon. She carries very little extra weight on her tall frame. At eighty years old, the lack of wrinkles on her face is stunning.

We sit at a table halfway between the kitchen and a living room that is straight out of *Home and Garden* magazine. The house is well-decorated, spotlessly clean, and uncluttered. A black and brown long-haired dachshund paces back and forth at my feet, eyeing me warily. I ask Mary if she would mind turning down the television. She apologizes as she picks up the remote control.

"My mother told me when you get up in the morning, turn all the TVs on for noise in the house," she explains. "If I hear something I'm interested in, I'll sit down and watch it, but usually I end up taking Cocoa for a walk. I've had three children and two husbands, and there was always something going on in the house. The TV is a big comfort to me."

The sudden silence seems heavy as Mary gets back to her story.

"We were married for ten and a half years. Richard was diagnosed two years ago, when we moved here. He was just not able to function anymore. I found out the bills weren't being paid. He hadn't written a check in two years. I started getting notices from the IRS and from the insurance companies. He always paid the bills. When I asked him about it, he said, 'Well, why don't you write the check?'

"That was very uncharacteristic. He kept a book with everything in it, every account. Everything was on its own line, then all of a sudden it wasn't. He just didn't want to think about anything like that.

"This is the economic side of Alzheimer's," Mary says, and I now know why she approached me after a caregivers' meeting and whispered, "They said I should talk to you."

She tells me, "We had a house in Miami that hadn't been sold. He kept turning down the offers. He wanted to keep his money like a tight fist, held close." She demonstrates her words as she speaks them.

"We have a wonderful neighborhood, and people come around to visit." She sweeps an arm toward the kitchen. "But one day, Richard sat right there at the stool by the island and he told the neighbor across the street, 'I'm going to put her ass on the street in the morning.'"

The words seem out of place coming from Mary's mouth. I ask if this was typical of Richard's language, and she shakes her head with a shudder.

"We had a wonderful relationship. He took me around the world. He was an airline pilot. We could go anywhere first class, and we did so for almost ten years. He would never have said anything like that. It wasn't his nature to talk like that to me, but he was like that with his first wife. I suppose that side of him came out with the Alzheimer's.

"My daughter reminded me that my mother had dementia, and that her personality changed. She would talk dirty when she never talked like that before. My grandmother had it, too, so I thought I was the one that was going to get it.

"I didn't care for the mean streak," Mary says, "but the main issue with my mother and with Richard is that they quit paying the bills. As I said, my husband was an airline pilot. They all had a checklist. He always paid the bills. Then I realized that he wasn't paying them. When he couldn't write checks, I did have some control, but I don't own this house. This house is in the trust, and the trust goes to his daughter and grandchildren. "

I ask Mary to tell me what happens now.

She holds her head high and says, "I'm eighty years old, and I'm left here without a roof over my head.

"A lot of people don't realize what they face right at the end," she explains. "It's very difficult when another family's involved. I should have made sure that I had a claim on this house. I should have broached that to him, but I really didn't know. The house is completely in his name, and his daughter and grandchildren get the house.

"When we married, I paid for half of our house in Miami and he paid half. Our prenuptial agreement read that each of us could stay in that house five years. After five years either of us could buy out the heirs or sell it. That was okay with me. It was a big house. I would not have stayed there.

"He wanted to move up here, and I did not want to come. We had a verbal agreement that if I came up here I would get the house, but I never had it in writing. That's the bottom line. His lawyer kept calling him and saying we had to redo his trust fund and everything, but with the dementia Richard kept saying, 'I'll do that tomorrow.' He kept putting it off. All I was trying to do was keep him alive. He had nine doctors. That's what we did. We went from one doctor to the other.

"I can't afford to buy this house and keep it up," she says. "I'm trying to get to stay here for five years, because that's what was in our prenup, but that applied only to the house in Miami. I didn't realize it didn't come up here."

She sums up the whole situation with a shrug. "It's a big kettle of fish."

I ask if she and her husband ever discussed his dementia.

"I don't think he ever faced his diagnosis. I asked the neurologist one time when we were walking out of the office if he had actually diagnosed him with dementia, and his answer was, 'Can't you tell?'

"It's a terrible disease. It's fine for the person that has it because they have no stress. Richard didn't have any. He wasn't worried about anything. He did not even complain about me driving the car. I thought that might be a problem. I said, 'You're driving me crazy. I'm going to drive the car.' Then, if I'd go over the speed limit, I'd hear 'Tsk, tsk, tsk,' but he didn't fight me.

"My friend Frances' husband Bill has Alzheimer's, and he is completely happy as long as he has his Chardonnay. Richard wanted his scotch and soda. I'd give it to him at five o'clock, then he wanted it at four. Did I give in and give it to him?" She throws her hands out. "Of course! What else is he going to do? He's not driving. They tell us in the group that you have to be careful with the drinking. They get mean and they don't want to go to bed. Alcohol can make them a little bit violent, but all he wanted was one.

"Caregivers have to have help. That's the first thing I would tell anyone. You can't do it by yourself. You can't leave them. I know Richard would not have left home, but he didn't like it when I left. When I got home he would say, 'You've been gone for two hours! Where have you been?' and I'd only been gone an hour. Time doesn't mean much to an Alzheimer's patient.

"After he died, I was at the cash register at a store, and I kept looking at my watch. The cashier said, 'Do you have an appointment?' and I said, 'No, it's just that I never stayed away more than an hour.'"

Mary looks around the empty house and says, "It's very hard for me to realize that I don't have to come home."

Cocoa sits at Mary's feet looking up at her with sad eyes.

"I had to have somebody come in at night when Richard was sick," she says, "because he was up every one to two hours. Everybody was telling me my health was going. He'd come in here and sit in his chair. I'd lie down on the sofa so I could watch him, because he fell a lot. I called 911 I don't know how many times. That's when I got the night nurse to come. Then I went to somebody in the daytime, too. I might have had an hour between the shifts when I was on my own.

"Toward the end he started sleeping a lot. That's a sign that your organs are shutting down. Have you ever heard of anyone dying of Alzheimer's?" she asks. "It's always something else. My mother had an aneurism.

"With my husband, I accepted his dying. I lost my first husband with throat cancer, so I'd been through it before. I could see when he was sleeping a lot that that was an indication. It happened in three days."

She snaps her fingers and says, "He went like that. People can live with Alzheimer's for years, but all of a sudden he started going downhill. I think it was the caregiver who alerted hospice, because they called me; I didn't call them. When the nurse said he had 24-48 hours, I couldn't believe it. In fact, I asked the nurse, 'When's he going to wake up? And she said, 'He's not going to wake up.' It's like a knife going through you."

Mary's composure begins to crack.

"I called his daughter. She and his son-in-law came in and took over the house completely with their children. They went through everything—files, cabinets . . . everything. And he could hear, you know? He couldn't speak, but he could hear.

"His daughter came in the door and looked at the nurse and said, 'I've been on the computer, and you're giving him the wrong medication.'"

Mary's words pick up speed as she relives the emotional last few days of her husband's life.

"They put me to bed that night. His daughter slept on the sofa, and she told the night nurse that she wanted his medication cut in half. She wanted him awakened, but he was in La La land."

She is crying now as she says, "When he died, his granddaughter stood over there telling everybody that she'd lost her grandfather, and I said, 'Honey, I have lost my husband!'"

Tears run down Mary's cheeks. "She told everybody I married him for his money, and I'm not getting a nickel!"

Her voice trails off while she dabs carefully at her face. When she speaks again, Mary's voice is tight. The words she spits out are like bullets that stun: "*I hate that little bitch.*"

In the seconds that follow, I expect to hear a hint of remorse for her outburst, but there is none.

"That girl was so bad to me the whole time I was married to him, but their grandmother—Richard's first wife—died, you know, and I'd been looking after him."

She stares out the window and slowly her jaw relaxes. "He had lost his wife with cancer, and I lost my husband the same way. We had ten wonderful years together. We really did.

"It's tough when you have a second family. That's the worst. With my first husband, my family was there, and with this one . . . ."

Mary returns now to the reason she wanted her story to be told.

"People need to know that when their spouses go down with this, the finances go out the window as far as they're concerned. Don't assume the bills are going to get paid, because they don't pay them. I'm eighty years old, and I don't want to move."

She reaches down and pats Cocoa on the head as she scans her eyes around the room.

"I'm a person that likes to know what's going to happen tomorrow. I like to see things in writing," Mary says, "and this I can't do right now."

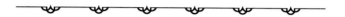

"How are you doing, Helen?" Judy asks a plump woman who has dark circles under her eyes as if her makeup has smeared.

"Not so good," she admits. "I've been trying to sort out the mess of papers in John's office, and I'm not getting anywhere." She runs a hand through her hair. "I feel so overwhelmed . . . . I'm almost at my wit's end."

"Call Brenda Lee," another woman offers.

Helen stares at the table. "I thought I could do this on my own."

"Brenda Lee is wonderful," Judy tells her. "She'll take care of you. Don't worry about it. You have enough to worry about."

Helen's tablemate leans close and says, "I have her card. I'll give it to you after the meeting."

10

PROPER PRIOR PLANNING

FINANCIAL ADVISOR BRENDA LEE RAY is used to going into people's houses to conduct her business. She appears confident and right at home as she steps into my house. She is attired professionally in a black dress with tan polka dots. Pearl earrings flank her attractive oval face. At thirty-something, she is far younger than most of her clients. She wears her blondish-brown hair long, and it suits her well.

We settle on my couch and she crosses her legs. She looks me right in the eye and sits tall. There is no slouching here. Instead, she radiates positive energy to the point of effervescence.

I study the logo on her business card, which reads, *"American Senior Financial."* Brenda Lee explains, "What my company does is help people protect their assets from nursing home expenses." Her head bobbles a bit from side to side, then she adds, "and assisted living and home care, too, but mostly nursing homes, because that's the biggest expense.

"We often deal with people pre-crisis, and that's what we call preplanning—just making sure they know what assets they have and where their assets are located. A lot of times they don't know. Maybe the person they're with is already starting to decline, memory-wise, and they haven't been brought up to speed yet about their financial situation. That's so common—that either he or she handled everything and didn't tell their partner what was going on.

"So, I go into people's homes, and it's like a puzzle. In order for me to advise them what to do, we have to first figure out what they have, asset-wise." Brenda Lee speaks animatedly with her hands as she says, "Maybe they have a life insurance policy that they bought back in 1961. They don't get statements anymore, and they've retired, and they've moved. It was a paid-up policy, so they never worried about it. So I have them sign an authorization to release information to me.

"We'll send off for the policy information, and we may find that it has $30,000 dollars in cash value, and the beneficiary listed is wrong. Maybe their children were too young when they first got it, so they only listed the wife as the beneficiary, and they had nobody listed as secondary. So I help them fix all that. That's what we can do in the preplanning stages. We just bring it all together: We figure out what they have and what money they should use first if they need to plan for care."

Brenda Lee says the problems arise when people don't take advantage of preplanning. She recalls helping Judy Simms when her husband Chuck was admitted to Arbor Village.

"I went there and Judy was so overwhelmed." She shakes her head. "And there are so many people like her. They have paper everywhere. They are so overwhelmed with the mental side of dealing with their situation that they can't keep up with anything else. So I went to Judy's house, and I took out bags of papers." She rolls her eyes.

"In fact, Judy still has grocery bags at my office," Brenda says, laughing. "She had stacks of papers everywhere. She was always doing things for everyone else, and she had no time, but I find that a lot."

She confirms that her company is not unique. "There are companies like this all over the country. What we do is considered Medicaid planning, and there are also attorneys who specialize in Medicaid laws."

She is careful to differentiate between Medicaid and Medicare. "Medicare applies to people age sixty-five and over. Part A of Medicare is their health insurance. They obtain that when they're sixty-five or disabled. We're all going to have that, hopefully. Part B we have to pay a little bit for. Part A covers hospitalizations, and Part B covers doctors. That's the easiest way to think of it.

"Medicaid is basically public assistance for people that can't afford health care. For instance, if somebody wants to qualify for Medicaid in a nursing facility, they have to be disabled, and Alzheimer's meets that qualification.

"The way it works for someone with Alzheimer's is that Medicare pays for skilled rehabilitation in a nursing facility for up to 100 days if the person had a three-day prior stay in a hospital. I have a lady right now whose mom needs care badly, but she can't get any Medicare coverage if she didn't go to a hospital for three days prior. So with Alzheimer's, how are you getting to the hospital? They have to go in for some other condition. Do you see what I'm saying?

"The thing is, once they're in the facility, if they need to stay long-term, the facility needs to keep their people who came in for rehab first. So that's the easiest way to get in."

She recaps the rules: "You have to be 65 to get Medicare. So, if you go to the hospital for three days for a fall or something, now you're sent to a rehab facility. Medicare will cover days one through twenty at one hundred percent. For days twenty-one up to one hundred, Medicare will cover all but a hundred and fifty dollars a day. If you have a secondary insurance or an HMO, some of those pick up that extra expense. Then, after a hundred days, the person goes private pay, and right now the nursing facilities in this area range from two hundred and ten, to two hundred and fifty dollars a day."

She makes an apologetic face, as if she is the one responsible for the high cost.

"That's where Medicaid can help, but only if you qualify for it." Brenda Lee looks up while considering the best way to explain the rules.

"Okay, let's say that, God forbid, you popped your husband in a nursing home." Again, she looks sorry. "You would be allowed to have only $109,560 dollars in assets. So, basically, you're not eligible for Medicaid until you spend down to this amount. And when I say 'spend down,' I mean private pay the care until you're down to $109,560 dollars."

She is quick to point out that things are not as bad as they sound. "In Florida your home is excluded as an asset, because Florida is a homestead state. That's a little different in some states. In some states they do the fifty-fifty rule, so you're allowed to have so many assets, but whatever you have, fifty percent would be yours and fifty percent your spouse's. In Florida, they allow the spouse at home to have a hundred and nine thousand dollars. So we would take your husband's name off your assets, because he's the one who needs care."

She crooks a finger and says, "You can't give away money, because Medicaid looks back five years on gifts, no matter where you live in the country. So, if you give away money, you have to do it more than five years in advance. In Florida, for instance, a lot of people have retirement accounts. Florida is an income-first state, and I've had so many people that I meet with tell me, 'I cashed out my IRA so I could get it in my name only.'" She lowers her voice to show how her clients think they did something clever.

"And I say, 'No! The IRA could be excluded. If it's generating income, we can exclude it as an asset!' So if you cash out a two hundred thousand dollar IRA, you just took something that was protected and made it an asset."

She shakes her head. "People don't know. I've spoken to Alzheimer's support groups, and they have so many people that say, 'Well, so and so told me to do this,' or, 'I did this, and you should do that.' Then I meet with them and I say, 'No, no, no, you don't have to do that!'" Her voice is gentle and filled with concern.

"They say, 'Medicaid will take my home. They'll take my car.' And I say, 'No, they don't. They don't take anything. They just don't give you benefits until your assets are down to these limits.' But people get scared."

She stresses the point: "They're not going to take anything.

"The problem in Florida, especially, is that people move here from all over the country, and the rules are different in every state. So I hear a lot of things like, 'Well, my mom was in a nursing home, and this is what happened in Connecticut,' or 'New York,' and the rules were different. It's very state-specific, and there's always somebody telling me things the neighbor down the street said, or the plumber, or the man that laid their floor . . . ."

She shudders.

"Those people may come from a different state, and they may not understand how Florida Medicaid works. So, you should inquire with a knowledgeable source right away, before you change anything. Once you cash out that IRA, for example . . . . If you were to do that, and I catch it within sixty days, you can put it back, but after that, I can't do anything. It's an asset then, so it's really important to get financial advice in advance from someone who understands Medicaid."

"I'll see these people sometimes who have been told by their financial advisor, 'Well, you're just going to have to spend some of your assets to get down to the hundred and nine thousand dollars, so you should start paying for the care until then.'" She throws her hands out in frustration with advisors who do their clients no favors, and says, "There are options available.

"We show people there are ways to legally protect their assets that exceed the hundred and nine thousand dollars. For instance, like I said, in Florida their home is excluded. Their car is excluded. The personal effects in the home are excluded. They can have life insurance, as long as the cash value doesn't exceed twenty-five hundred dollars. They can also have prepaid burial arrangements, and there are other ways to protect the assets. But again, the problem is that regulations vary state to state, so you need to check on your state laws. There are states that are more strict than others.

"In a lot of states the home isn't protected. These people work their whole lives and save. In some states, when they die, the home is subject to a state recovery, meaning that once the proceeds come out, Medicaid has to be reimbursed. So Florida is a good state to go to a nursing home in," she says, smiling.

"If someone just put their spouse in a home and they didn't do any preplanning, they're now in a crisis. They're like, 'Uh oh, we're going to start incurring seven thousand dollars a month now in expenses,' depending on their prescriptions and other things. That's when we try to calm them down. We file the application with Medicaid for them." Brenda Lee stresses, "We explain to Medicaid what we did with every penny—whether we moved it to the spouse, or what we did with it. And then we serve as the designated representative and take care of all the paperwork for them. They don't even talk to Medicaid. We do it all."

It is clear that Brenda Lee cares about people, and this explains how she got into her current line of work.

"I started in this business by selling nursing home insurance. I was in the top ten in the whole country. This was back when long-term care insurance was new. There were people who might have had, say, a mini-stroke, and if they weren't in perfect health, they couldn't get the long-term insurance. That's when my wheels started turning, and I was like, 'Hmmm . . . . What do they do if they can't get it?'"

Speaking as she would about her own parents, Brenda Lee says, "They worked their whole lives. They tried to get the insurance once it became available, but they already had a health problem. What do they do now? Nothing. What do they do? And that's when I started doing the Medicaid planning, and I've been doing that for seven years now.

"I made less money when I started doing this. It started with just me and one other person. I'm finally getting to a point where I'm making more now. I didn't know this service existed, but I just felt it was so unfair that these people would try to get insurance when it was new. They'd had a little mishap in their health that a lot of people in their seventies have, and they couldn't get insurance, and now they had to spend their money! I knew what nursing homes cost, and I knew there had to be another way. That's when I started researching it."

She sticks her chin out. "The rich people have been protecting their money for a very, very long time. There's no reason that the middle class average person can't do it, too.

"Medicaid is not for the rich, but if somebody has a decent amount of money, say a few hundred thousand, but the wife is young and she's not going to get a pension, we can foresee that she's going to need more money. She's not going to make it. So we're going to be as creative as possible to protect that.

"Preplanning is the most important thing. It's so important to know what you can do to protect your assets. That's a big concern for couples, because, say you have a husband and wife . . . the wife is sixty-two and the husband is seventy-five, and you put him into a facility. Say they have three hundred thousand dollars that they've saved together over the years. She was a stay-at-home mom, and the only income she has is Social Security of maybe seven hundred and sixty dollars a month. It's low because she's drawing a portion of her husband's, because she stayed home and took care of the children.

"And now she places him in a facility. She has to private pay the costs until her assets are down to one hundred and nine thousand dollars. Then, when she does private pay down to a hundred and nine thousand, when we go to obtain Medicaid benefits, then her husband's income may all have to go to the facility's monthly bill, because she still has to pay something, even though she's on Medicaid.

"There is a spousal diversion. Medicaid does let you keep a portion of your husband's income, but maybe now she gets a thousand dollars of her husband's income. The other two thousand dollars is going to the facility. So now she only has a hundred and nine thousand to last the rest of her life, and she's only sixty-two! Then she realizes that her husband, when he retired, instead of taking a spousal benefit on his pension, he took the greater amount so that they could live more comfortably, not realizing that when he dies, she gets none of his income."

Brenda Lee's eyes tear up as she paints this picture. It is obvious that this is not just a hypothetical scenario, but one that she has seen time and time again.

"Even if you obtain Medicaid, you will probably have to give up a portion of your income to the facility—and that's in every state of the country. Every spouse should know what their income is going to look like if they lose their loved one, regardless of just needing care. Most of the women I meet with don't know what they would get from their husband's pension if he died. They just don't know. And in the age group I'm working with, most of them stayed home. They don't get a pension.

"If you find out that your partner has Alzheimer's," Brenda Lee advises, "contact a knowledgeable source—someone that specializes in dealing with the Medicaid office. It could be an attorney, or someone who offers my services. Ask questions, and if you don't get the answer you want, ask someone else.

"The family I met with this morning has been private-paying the nursing home bill for two years. They didn't know that someone like me existed. It's not the nursing home's job to advise people in these matters. They can't give insurance advice, financial advice, or tax advice. I can't give legal advice or tax advice either, because I'm not an attorney or a CPA, but there are many things we can do that are allowable."

To find advisors who do what she does, Brenda suggests a search on the Internet for "Medicaid protections."

"I've had several people whose financial advisor told them that there was nothing they could do but private-pay. They've been with that guy for twenty-five years, and they trust him wholeheartedly. He didn't do anything wrong. He just didn't know! He doesn't do Medicaid. Do you see what I'm saying? But they didn't search anywhere else, because they see Billy that they've been going to for twenty years, and he told them, so that must be what the rules are."

She lets her hands flop onto the couch. Her frustration is palpable.

"A lot of people here in Florida kept their old financial advisor, or CPA, or attorney from out of state, and the rules are different here. They're not the same. Their advisors are not doing it intentionally. They just don't know the rules. So keep looking. You'll know when you've found the right answer. Then, when you find someone who gives you an answer you want, double-check them! Ask for references. Ask what type of dealings they have with the local Medicaid office. Usually, elder-law attorneys are a great place to start. They can be very helpful."

Brenda Lee winces. "I'm nervous that people are going to read this, and it's going to be just like when their neighbor tells them to do something. I would feel horrible if people did something that wasn't true in their state, so they need to check their state rules.

"We had one of my clients all set for Medicaid here at Arbor Village. He called us one day and said, 'They're not giving Medicaid to her in Maryland.' Maryland is an asset-first state, so the IRA isn't protected there. I said, 'Okay, was someone going to tell us this?' She moved up there with her daughter. That's when they called us and said, 'It doesn't appear she's getting Medicaid there. What you did here didn't work.' I said, 'You should have called us before you moved her, because the rules are different.' Now, she's there."

Brenda Lee shakes her head. "It's crazy. It really is."

"Alzheimer's is the saddest one out of all the illnesses we deal with because the stay in a nursing home is longer," she says. "They're physically fine. It's just mental, so they're happier. They have not a care in the world, and I firmly believe stress is a big ailment causer. If you don't have a care in a world, you could live a long time.

"I think about that myself a lot," Brenda Lee says as she gazes around the room. "You see that they don't have a lot of in-depth thoughts. I don't know what they're thinking about, but they're physically fine. Some of them used to have high blood pressure for years, and now they have Alzheimer's, and they don't need blood pressure medication!"

She cocks her head and says, "You are what you think about.

"I don't pretend to know a lot about Alzheimer's, but one thing I know is that when I get a call for somebody about preplanning, I tell them to do this, and this, and this, and they say, 'Well, it should be a couple of years before I place him or her.' Then they have a fall or something and it just drives them into high gear. I don't know why, but it always happens. I'll ask them, 'How did this happen so quickly?' Almost always they say they broke a shoulder or a hip or something. They have that one little mishap, and pshhhhhhh—"

She moves her hand as if sliding down a hill. And with a shake of her head, she adds, "And it's a long stay."

"Helping people protect their assets is my thing," Brenda Lee states with authority, then her voice softens.

"I'm going to start a not-for-profit organization. I have six people that work at my office with me, and right now I can't take the time to help these people like I want. Until I get that up and going, I keep telling people, 'Do this planning while you're healthy and you can make the decisions, while you're thinking clearly.

"Do it all in advance," she advises, "and stash it away somewhere."

And then, with a sparkle in her warm, dark eyes, Brenda Lee Ray shares her number one advice for people of any age: "Plan for the worst, and hope for the best."

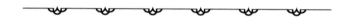

Judy moves on to a man in a maroon polo shirt. The pocket bears the logo of a home health care company. "Okay," she says, "I'm going to introduce Roy for a minute. He has become like family. He kept saying, 'Judy, I want to help, I want to help, I want to help.' Well, this man helped at the square on the night we had the memorial service. He's done all kinds of things behind the scenes. He's just always there for us. So, I invited him to sit in today so that you all could see what a really nice family member we have. He's truly a caring man."

She looks Roy in the eyes and tells him, "I've taken your turn and talked for you today, okay?"

It is clear that Judy wants to give Roy public thanks without giving the appearance of endorsing any one business.

Roy returns her smile. "Okay."

A woman three seats to Roy's right leans in and says,

"I'm sorry. Does he have a last name? And does he have a card?"

Judy jumps in. "He has a card, and if you go right out on the table in the hallway, there's a flyer for his company, but we're not soliciting. There are all sorts of home health care companies out there, but those who come and work with us are special." She flashes Roy an appreciative smile.

Roy can't sit quietly. "My grandfather was diagnosed with Alzheimer's," he says, "and I spent the majority of my childhood with him." Roy's accent places that childhood somewhere around North Carolina.

"He was the pillar in my life, and I watched my pillar deteriorate to a state that it's hard to put my mind around. It was crushing to me. For six years my family took care of my grandfather in our living room in a hospital bed, with no outside help whatsoever. We had no clue that there was any help available to us, or anything called 'home health care.' There was absolutely nothing offered to us except hospice when it got to that point.

"A year ago I was led to Miss Judy, and as I believe in fate very much, I knew I'd kind of found my calling. Since then, I have established my home health care company with one hundred percent support from my wife. We run this agency with passion for the people that we meet because of what we've been through."

He makes sure to add, "It's not just, 'Oh, I'm a business. Come see us and spend money with us.' I think we come across as genuine, because it comes from our heart. I can relate to each and every one of you in this room, because I've seen the highs, and I've seen the valleys. Some of them were lower than you can imagine, and every once in a while a peak would stand out as a bright star."

Roy's eyes rove around the room, touching everyone

present as he advises, "Cherish every single minute of it. Some of those will turn out to be your very best memories."

"Thank you," Judy says. She seems a bit uncomfortable that he has spoken about his business, but she appears pleased, nonetheless, with his heartfelt words.

"Thank you for allowing me to come here," Roy replies. "I truly feel at home."

"You're family," Judy beams, and adds a quick, "Don't cry, Roy."

"I won't," he says, and the group laughs as Roy wipes a very real tear.

11

WITH GOD'S HELP

I ARRIVE AT THE HOME OF BILL AND FRANCES FROST. The woman who opens the door wearing a pair of white shorts and a bright print top is much younger than I expected. She is talking on the phone and moves it away from her lips to mouth the words, *"I'm the caregiver."* She then motions me into the house with a nod of her head.

A man about five-foot-seven with wire-rimmed glasses and a full head of gray hair wanders into the entry hall. Seeing me, he gives a cheery "Hello." I introduce myself, and he tells me his name is Bill. He doesn't ask why I am there. He simply stands in the hallway and smiles pleasantly.

The caregiver, who has taken her phone conversation into the open kitchen to my left, motions Bill and me toward the living room beyond.

I take a seat in an armchair while Bill settles onto an adjacent sofa. We have an easy chat in which I ask all of the questions. He tells me that he used to be an airline pilot. I ask what airline he flew for, and we go on to discuss inter-airline competition. Other than the brevity of his contributions to the conversation, it is not readily apparent that Bill has Alzheimer's.

Bill's wife Frances enters the house from the garage. Her outfit is cheery and youthful: black Capri pants and a pink top with a matching print blouse over it. She takes the empty chair next to mine, not bothering to remove her sporty pink cap.

When I compliment her on the hat, she reaches up and runs her fingers through the blond hair that peeks out from under the visor. "It's a necessity," she says. Only now does it become apparent that the hair is a wig—sewn under the brim of the cap.

"I'm going through chemotherapy for breast cancer," she says, which explains why she looks so tired. "I lost my hair after the first treatment two months ago. I really haven't looked at it. I try not to."

Everything about Frances is warm and soft—her voice, her eyes, and even her smile, as she discusses her baldness.

Bill sits on the couch across from us, still smiling pleasantly. He has yet to ask who I am or why I am there. I ask Frances if we can talk freely.

She studies Bill for a moment, then says softly, "Maybe he should go." In a louder voice she says to her husband, "Do you want to go for an ice cream?"

He perks up and says, "Sure!" No questions asked.

Frances calls over to the caregiver, who is off the phone now. "Sheryl, would you like to take Bill for some ice cream?"

"That sounds good," Sheryl replies, without missing a beat. "Come on, Bill, let's go out."

He rises from the couch, and as he walks toward the door, Bill says cheerfully, "I don't know why I need ice cream, but it looks like we're going!"

Frances watches until he is out the door, then says, "He was diagnosed officially six years ago, but of course we noticed it before that. The last time his neurologist ran the tests, she said he had gone down two points. I don't know what that means, exactly, but he has deteriorated in the last year or so. He's definitely not in the 'severe' category . . . moderate-plus, maybe."

She is wearing a necklace with a snazzy silver star on the chain. She fingers the star now as she relates, "The other day we were sitting at the counter having lunch, and Bill said, 'Do you remember my mom and dad's names? I don't remember.' Of course, I started crying," she says, and her eyes fill now as she retells the story. "It's just so sad when that happens."

I ask about the caregiver.

"Sheryl started about a year ago," Frances says, "and she is very good with him. She's usually the one that comes, and we prefer her. Fortunately, we have long-term care insurance. I really encourage people to get that. Only seven percent of the population has it, you know, and it's a blessing, blessing, blessing." She shakes her head as if she can't imagine life without it.

"Sheryl comes three or four days a week for seven hours. She's here from nine-thirty to four-thirty or ten to five. Whatever I want. Without a caregiver, I can only leave Bill alone for an hour, maybe. Sometimes on Sunday I go to church. That may be for an hour and a half, but he gets very anxious. When I get home he says, 'I was worried about you.' He gets paranoid, which is very common. He thinks people are back here watching us." She points toward the back yard. "And he always wants to shut the blinds.

"He doesn't know why the caregiver is here," Frances admits. "He'll say, 'When is our guest leaving?' Sometimes Sheryl will spend the night if we're doing back-to-back days, because she lives an hour or so away, and she doesn't charge us for that."

She explains that Sheryl has a family of her own, but that she and her husband own the home care company. "We're lucky to have her. I don't know how people do it without help. It's unbelievable, the stress." She makes a guilty face. "I had a little meltdown yesterday."

I ask her to explain what constitutes a meltdown.

She gives a weak smile. "I mean that I had no patience with him. I say things that are not real nice sometimes. Yesterday we went to the town square. He likes to go there. Thank God for the music," she interjects. "That saves me. I can sit there for an hour and a half without answering all the questions.

"But yesterday, we came home from the square, and he expects to have his food right there. I said, 'No, we're going to sit on the patio and turn the music on while dinner's in the oven.' So, every few minutes he asked, 'When are we going to eat? What time are we going to eat?' But what happens is, if we eat, he wants to go right to bed, and he wants me to go with him. So, if we eat at six o'clock, he's ready to go to bed at six-thirty or seven.

"I don't usually give in until about eight o'clock; then I'll go in with him and watch television. But yesterday he said, 'Why are you so mad at me?' and I'm going, 'I don't know! I'm just pissed off,' and I mean, I was slamming doors and doing things I shouldn't have. Then you lie in bed feeling guilty that you were upset with him.'"

She does, indeed, look guilty.

"We were in Miami when he was diagnosed," she says. "He's the one that wanted to go to the doctor. He just thought he was having memory loss. We're talking seven years ago. And sure enough, when we got there, he couldn't answer the questions, like how to count backwards, or where he lived. See, right now he doesn't know this address, but he knows to pull out a little card with the address on it. He doesn't know the kids' names, either. He'll say, 'How many kids do we have?' and we have three."

She tells me that Bill is seventy-seven, and confirms that he was an airline pilot. I tell her that we chatted about his career and that Bill told me he flew for Delta.

Frances gapes in surprise. "He knew that?" She shakes her head with wonder.

"Things come and go," she says. "There are times when you think, 'How in the world did he remember that?' And there are times when his memory is totally gone." She leans her head back, then says, "You just don't know what they're thinking. He pretends to read the paper. I think it's so cute. He sits there all morning reading it. I'll ask him something about what he's reading, and he has no clue."

She remarks that their days are not without humor.

"The other day we went to my sister's house. She lives about ten minutes from here. My niece is gay, and we went over to meet her new friend." Frances makes little quotation marks with her fingers as she says the word "friend."

"So we visited, and we had a snack, and of course the 'friend' was very masculine. As we drove away, Bill looked at me and he said, just as serious as can be, 'I don't understand why that man has tits!'"

We laugh, and she says, "He comes up with stuff like that every now and then.

"If you're not exposed to Alzheimer's, you're like, 'Oh, Alzheimer's . . . . Reagan had that, right?' I didn't understand it a lot when Bill first got it. I think when I really got concerned that something was wrong was this one day when he didn't come back from the barber shop. I got worried that he was gone so long. He finally came home and he said, 'I couldn't find my way home.' We had lived in the same house for thirty-seven years! That's the moment I thought, 'We've got a serious problem here.' So then I started not letting him go out alone so much."

She recalls a time when someone on the television was talking about Alzheimer's. "Bill said, 'You know, I think that's what I have,' but that's the only time he's mentioned it.

"He doesn't even know what Alzheimer's is. He'll say, 'You know, I really can't remember things anymore,' and I'll say, 'Honey, you have a problem,' and he'll say, 'Well, wait 'til you get to be my age!'"

She laughs, because she is seventy-five years old—just two years younger than her husband.

"I can see him getting worse. He walks around the house shaving, and this morning he said, 'I found this in the garage.' He had his razor in his hand. He said, 'Does it go over there?' and he pointed to where the telephone goes. So you can tell it's getting worse. Fortunately he doesn't wander off down the street." She adds a quick, "So far . . . ."

"He's really better than some people you hear about," she says in Bill's defense. "I have to make sure he bathes properly, but he gets in the shower and attempts to clean himself. He's not real incompetent yet, but I know it's going to get worse."

Frances fingers her necklace again.

"I still feel bad about my little meltdown, but . . . well . . . I've been a bit depressed because of all of this," she points at her wig, then runs her hands down the rest of her body.

"I've not been well for about three years," she explains. "Before my cancer, I had arterial bypasses in both legs." She pulls up one leg of her Capri pants to reveal a shockingly long scar that begins five inches below the knee and disappears beneath the black cloth.

"It's twenty-five inches," she says. "It goes all the way to my abdomen. They took a vein and made an artery out of it. I had PAD—Peripheral Arterial Disease—and the artery in my leg was totally blocked. I could not walk. My father had the same disease. He actually lost his leg from it, so that scared me.

"I had my surgery in February of last year. It was horrible, and to deal with that at the same time as dealing with Bill . . . . It was just awful."

I remark that the scar is well healed.

"Didn't they do a wonderful job?" she says. "Oh—I'm not supposed to cross my legs!" She puts both feet flat on the floor, and flashes another guilty smile. "The doctors didn't want to do this. It's a very serious operation, but I said, 'You know what? I don't want to live this way.'"

She leans back into the chair, propped like a rag doll against the cushion, and announces, "Nine months later, they diagnosed me with cancer. I was so wrapped up in caring for Bill that I didn't take care of myself. I think I wanted to deny there was a problem, because I could definitely feel a lump in my breast for quite a long time.

"The really sad thing is not having support from Bill. He has no clue what I'm going through. No clue. He asks me, 'Why don't you have hair? Why did they shave your head? Why are they doing this to you?' I tell him, 'I have cancer,' but five minutes later he'll ask me again. When I had to have a mastectomy, he seemed to understand that more than the hair loss, for some reason.

"That was six months ago, so I had two major surgeries in the same year, plus I had a stent put in my heart." She turns both palms upward as if to say, *What're you going to do?*

"I have to fight the depression," Frances admits. "I have pity parties all the time. You know, 'Why don't I have hair? Poor me, I don't have any boobs . . . .' She makes a sad-clown face. 'Should I have reconstructive surgery?' I just don't know! It's totally frustrating not having Bill's support.

"Thank God for family and friends. My daughter and my daughter-in-law have been here for my operations and recoveries. My daughter-in-law actually came thirteen times in one year to help me. For the leg surgery, I was six days in the hospital, and Bill stayed with my daughter-in-law and son. For the mastectomy I was just in overnight." She flashes me a *"Can you believe that?"* look, then adds, "Sharon stayed here in the house with Bill that night."

She exhales slowly, then announces, "I don't cry a whole lot. I fill up pretty often, but I try not to cry. I think you're afraid to start. There for a while, I would get emotional when I went to church—when I was sitting there by myself—but I'm not going to let him take that away from me just because he gets worried while I'm gone. I need my church. Eventually I'm going to have to have someone come in on Sunday to be with him."

I ask her how she deals with the stress. She takes a moment to respond.

"Well, my support group is about it." She pauses, then adds, "And I have a couple of glasses of wine at night. That helps. Of course, he does, too. He likes his Chardonnay. People frown on it, but I think he sleeps better when he has a drink or two. Fortunately, that helps me to get some rest if he's sleeping."

She is quick to point out, "I don't let him have all he wants. I control it, and the doctor knows about it. I told her, 'You know, he's been enjoying his wine for a lot of years, and I see no reason why he can't have it.'"

She realizes she has gotten off track and says, "As for the support group, I really miss it when I don't go. It's phenomenal to be with other people who are in the same situation you're in. Sometimes you sit there and think, 'Oh, I'm not so bad off after all.' And sometimes you're worse off than somebody else, but it's a great way to talk and meet people.

"I saw an ad for the support group in the paper. I had gone to another one a while back, but it was so depressing that I stopped going. Maybe I didn't give it a chance," she admits, "but like I said, the new one is phenomenal."

She tilts her head as she reflects, "It might have been the timing of when I went to the first group. Maybe I wasn't ready for it." Now she nods. "I think it was me, and not the meeting. Absolutely. The timing wasn't right yet.

"I tried taking Bill and putting him in the respite care while I was in the meetings." She shakes her head as if that was not a good idea. "One time he sat next to somebody who was farther along than him, and he just didn't like it."

She tosses her hand out. "Why put myself through that if I have Sheryl to stay with him? I know it's good to get him out with the others in respite care, but we go out a lot with friends. Sometimes he wants to drink too much when we go out to dinner, but two is his limit. I don't want him to fall and hurt himself. The other couples we go out with don't have Alzheimer's. They're wonderful with him, they really are.

"I used to like to entertain. I have a very good friend . . . ." She points a finger, and says, "I think you interviewed her—Mary Baxter."

I confirm that I did interview Mary.

"I was actually friends with her husband Richard for sixty years before I met Mary. We were all in the same yacht club. I knew Richard before I knew Bill. They were both pilots, you know."

We talk for a few minutes about Mary's situation.

"It's gotten even worse since you talked to her," Frances says. "They're kicking her out. First Richard's children were going to let her stay there for a while, then they wanted all this money to write up a contract, so she chose not to do all that. She's moving out as we speak."

Frances shakes her head. "I just hope her story will keep other people from doing what she did. She didn't have the paperwork in order. I would have had more security. Now the kids and the lawyers are going to get it all. She's very bitter, and I don't blame her."

Frances makes an *"enough of that"* motion with her hands and gets back to discussing the ways she takes care of herself.

"I try to get out of the house when the caregiver is here."

She squints, then lowers her voice and says in a conspiratorial tone, "I go *shopping.*" Her whole demeanor changes as she says the word, and we laugh.

"Sometimes I go to see my sister. Usually I don't rush right out, though, because Sheryl is here for seven hours. I used to think, 'Seven hours! What am I going to do out all the time?' But I'm not usually gone the whole seven hours.

"Today I didn't even leave until noon. When she's here, she'll pick up, and clean, and wash his clothes, and fix his lunch. Sometimes she'll take him out to lunch, and she goes to Wal-Mart for me." Frances wrinkles her nose. "I hate to go there, but she'll take Bill and she makes him walk the whole store.

"Sheryl tried doing activities with him at first," she remembers. "I tried it, too—things like coloring and connect-the-dots, but he didn't like it. Now she'll have him water the plants or put the silverware away and fold napkins. Stuff like that."

Frances suddenly gets a devilish look on her face and confides, "Two weeks ago, I ran away from home for three days! I went with the girls." She gazes away for a moment, lost in the pleasant memory. "It was nice. We had a 'girl week,' and Bill was okay. Sheryl stayed with him. It eats away at the money we have allotted for home care, but you know what? We can't worry about that. Fortunately, we're in a good position financially with his pension, and thank God we had the long-term care insurance.

"We're very lucky to have the in-home care," Frances admits, "but if something happened to me, Bill would have to go in a home right away. Right now he's healthier than I am, and it used to be the other way around. When we moved up here five years ago, I took one prescription pill. I was so healthy; I walked three miles a day, five days a week, at least. I was doing that until the leg thing started. Now I can't even count all the pills.

"He used to have high blood pressure and high cholesterol, and he doesn't have any of that anymore. His blood pressure is unbelievably good. But if he got really, really bad, I don't think we'd do the full-time care here because of the stress on me.

"I think we're a couple of years out from putting him in a home—if I can hold on that long," she adds with a wince. "I'm sure I can," she says a half-beat later with more confidence. "It's just the stress and this chemo right now. I think I'm tired because I didn't sleep well last night. This is my bad week, because the chemo just wears you out. I had my treatment last Tuesday. It was my third one, and each time it's taken me about ten days to get over it."

She musters a smile. "Next week will be better. I have just one more treatment, then I have to do radiation five days a week for five or six weeks." She makes this matter-of-fact announcement as if she has steeled herself for the next round.

"Usually I'm a very up person," she says, as if she needs to make excuses, "but it's just this week that I don't feel good. I'll be over this in a few days . . . " she glances at the couch where Bill was seated when the interview began. "It's just kind of hard to stay 'up' with all that's going on.

"To me, the real Alzheimer's is not having the support of your spouse and knowing that it's not going to get better. There are always going to be bumps in the road that you can't share. It's just such a dreadful disease . . . the devastation to your family is very hard."

She confides, "I get the feeling our two sons are uncomfortable caring for their dad. We went down to see our son, and he watched Bill while we girls went shopping for a couple of hours. By the time we got back, he was totally overwhelmed," she says, describing her son, not her husband.

"He said to me, 'How do you stand this, Mom? How do you put up with him going in and out, opening and closing the garage door, asking questions all day? He asks the same questions over and over! How in the world do you stand it?'"

She gives a "*Welcome to my world*" look.

I ask her the same question her son asked her: How does she stand it?

Frances takes a deep breath, then replies softly, "With God's help." Tears flood her eyes, and she repeats, "With God's help. Absolutely. I pray every morning," she says, choking on the words. "I thank God every morning for my legs, then I think, 'Don't feel so sorry for yourself, because they've taken away parts of your body!' She puts a hand to her chest. "Actually, the hair thing was worse than this . . . and I had *really* nice hair. I'll show you."

She rises from her chair and crosses the living room. She picks up a framed photo from on top of the television set. "Everybody likes my wigs, but it was nice hair," she says with an embarrassed laugh as she hands me the picture.

It is a family photo in which Frances stands next to Bill, and indeed, she had very nice hair—blond, soft, and full.

"This was taken at our granddaughter's wedding," she explains, asking, "Aren't they a cute couple?" as she points to the bride and groom. "This was three years ago. Bill is smiling in that picture, but he didn't know what we were doing there."

She lowers herself into the chair and says, "Five years ago we had our fiftieth wedding anniversary party. He didn't know what was going on then, either. He kept asking, 'What are we doing here? Why are all these people here?' But I wanted a party, so we had one. I put him in his pilot's uniform. No one knew he was going to wear it except me. We walked down the aisle of a church, and we renewed our vows, and he just said, 'What are we doing here?'"

She takes the framed picture and sets it on the end table beside her.

"I'm sorry I was so down today," she apologizes needlessly, then says, "I just hope I sleep better tonight."

She glances at the wedding photo and smiles. "We're having a family reunion here in June, so that'll give me something to look forward to."

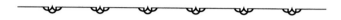

Judy Simms turns to her right and nods. "Ava?"

A tall woman in her seventies with dark hair and dark eyes nods back. She has an air of dignity and strength as she looks around the table at her fellow caregivers. "For some of you who might have missed the last few meetings," she says, "my stepson, who has durable power of attorney, arranged to pick up his dad for permanent residency with him and his wife as permanent caregivers."

She turns to her left and sends an appreciative smile to Judy. "I had my angels with me during the transition and afterwards. I had a biopsy the next day, and my friend Anita was there to pick me up. I spent Christmas day with my neighbors, and New Year's Day with my good support group friends, so I was surrounded by love the entire time. I have friends all over the United States, and ironically, every one of them called over the holiday season, as if they felt something was wrong. They were all in contact.

"With me, it's been a lot of 'Let go and let God,' and 'This too shall pass,' and emailing everybody when I'm down in the dumps. I think as a whole I've remained rather positive. I've learned that you can survive with support and love, and that there are many people with heavier burdens than I've had to go through.

"I'm still in our same home. His son took all of Andrew's belongings, so I could probably run a few bowling balls through the house, because half of the stuff's gone."

A woman across the room says, "Furniture and everything?"

"Yes. Yes," Judy answers for Ava. "I have to tell you that she was wonderful through all of this, and this was not something anybody wants to see. Let me tell you, this

was a tragedy happening. She was wonderful, and it went smoothly."

Ava sticks her thumb out in Judy's direction like a hitchhiker, saying, "Well, little Napoleon here helped . . . ."

The group erupts in laughter at the reference to Judy.

Judy waggles her shoulders and says, "But we did a good job, and I could see that when he was gone—and that was the hard part—I could see this 'lift' in Ava's spirits."

The group hums in understanding.

"The pain was there," Judy confirms, "but the lift, you could see it in her face. And then we went out to MacDonald's afterwards and had the most wonderful wrap! But she did well for what she was going through."

All heads turn back to Ava, who says, "I've had so many positive things come from all of this, that long term it's probably the best thing that could happen. His children are in denial. They certainly need to learn some lessons of life."

"Oh," drawls a woman four seats to Ava's right. "They'll learn . . . ."

12

THE MASTERFUL TEACHER

AVA BALDWIN HOLDS UP A CARDBOARD CUT-OUT of an acorn. A small orange pumpkin and a yellow leaf with glitter are glued on top. It is the kind of craft that a kindergartner would bring home for his mother to stick on the front of the fridge. No little fingers put the finishing touches on this ornament, but the gnarled hands of Ava's eighty-four-year-old husband, Andrew.

"This," she says wryly while looking at the artwork, "from a man who helped to design the skyline of a major US city."

Andrew crafted the acorn while attending respite care at a local church. The activities kept him and his friends who suffer from Alzheimer's "meaningfully engaged." It is not they who need the respite, however, but their caregivers. Their loved ones get the break they so badly need a few doors down the hall at their weekly support group meeting.

Ava sets the acorn on an end table in her recently rearranged living room. She picks up a white heart with several small pink hearts affixed to it. She turns it over in her fingers, fondling the edges, and says, "This was my treasure for Valentine's Day. He made it last year, but this year I had nothing. I had invited him to join me for dinner seven days beforehand, but they told me he already had plans."

"They" are Andrew's son and daughter-in-law. It has been two months since they took Andrew from the home he shared with Ava, his wife of ten years. She has only seen him once since then—but not at Christmas, not at New Year's, and not on her birthday in January. It has not been for lack of trying. She is now paying a lawyer to look into the visitation situation. In the meantime, the excuses keep coming from the rented home where Andrew is living with his son, just five miles away.

"We had hopes of doing extensive traveling when we married," she says, looking wistfully around the quiet house. "Eighteen months into the marriage I noticed that he seemed to be forgetting a lot of things. He wasn't paying bills, and we were getting second notices. Andrew is twelve years older than I am, so at first I attributed it to the age difference.

"A major indicator that something was wrong occurred when we went to visit his children. He thought he was going one direction, when he was actually going the opposite way. This was so unusual, because he knew all the best restaurants, hotels, and anything historical in the area. He was an encyclopedia of information. Many times we took side roads, and I'd say, 'I wonder what's down there?' and he'd say, 'Well, let's go see!'

"So, we were coming home, and I never double-checked his directions. We drove fifty miles out of town, and I could tell it wasn't the right highway. Then another time we went to visit his daughter, and she was giving him directions. He'd lived there all of his life. He worked there in construction and had been up and down the highway a thousand times. He didn't have a clue where he was, and he was going the opposite way of what she'd just told him at the breakfast table. This, and the frequency of his forgetting, alerted me to a real problem."

Ava explains that they consulted a family friend who was a pediatrician. "He sent Andrew to an internist, who conducted blood tests and a brain scan. The scan showed indicators of dementia. The doctor referred him to a neurologist, who diagnosed his condition as a mild case of Alzheimer's in the beginning stages. I had no idea then how deeply it would affect us."

She looks down at the pink hearts which now lie at her side.

"We were always very honest with each other. We would talk nonstop for hours. So we got to the house and I said, 'I think we need to discuss this.' He said, 'I will tell you how I feel about other things, but as far as I'm concerned, we're not going to discuss this with anyone.'

"It was like a book that would never be opened. Case closed. He is very mild-mannered and low key, but there was a finality to his statement. I said, 'There will be some day we have to discuss it,' and he said, 'We'll take it in stride.' That's one of his classic statements.

"I was so tied up at the time caring for my mother with a brain hemorrhage that I just left it alone. Knowing Andrew, if he didn't want to talk about it, that was his business. Then we moved to Florida, and immediately he began introducing himself by saying, 'I'm Andrew Baldwin. I have dementia.'

"I guess he grew comfortable with the fact that he had Alzheimer's, and he realized it was probably evident, because he would have to ask me what neighborhood we lived in, what was our address, and 'How old am I?' He camouflaged it very well in conversation, but he was cognizant that he could no longer remember facts.

"It probably affected me more than it did him. You see someone who has such knowledge and brilliance and ability who wants to please you and goes out of his way to do so. For our first date he booked the private dining room of Ruth's Chris Steakhouse. He would always do unique things for special occasions. That slowly diminished until he couldn't select a restaurant, and then he couldn't order from a menu, and then he couldn't distinguish what was on a plate. It got to the point where he would look at an omelet and toast and say, 'Is this food for me? What is that?'"

She sighs and shakes her head. "Here you have a man with such capacity—such presence—then all of a sudden he's like a three-year-old toddler, but a toddler is like a sponge trying to learn. Andrew is like a sponge that is drying out. That's what it does to the brain. It shrinks it."

She points a finger. "This is why support groups are so important. Hearing other people's stories prepares you for when the symptoms show up. One symptom I had a hard time dealing with was the layering of clothes. This past Easter I dressed him in blue slacks, a shirt, and a blazer. He had forgotten how to tie a tie, so he quit wearing them two years ago.

"That's very common," she says as an aside. "They change their habits because of not knowing how to do things. Two years ago he would come out with a black shoe, a brown shoe, his shirt on with the buttons in back, his pants on with the zipper in back, and different colored socks. So, by last Easter he could no longer dress himself. I always got him dressed completely. I zippered his fly and had to put his belt on. He would just put it over the loops or put every belt in the closet on, one on top of the other. Many times if I'd run to answer the phone, he'd have two belts on.

"That morning at Easter we were running late. We got to the church and went to the communion rail. I always had to tell him how to kneel, because he'd stand and look at me and wait. I'd take his hands and position them, or else he'd drink the whole chalice of wine. So I looked down, and there's another pair of cuffs sticking out from under his pant legs. He had gone to the laundry room and put them on over his dress pants. Had I not gone to the support group and known this kind of thing happened, it would have been a shocking experience."

She takes a deep breath. "That morning I was just annoyed with myself that I hadn't double-checked him. I felt I was to blame. He didn't know any better. You assume responsibility, and then you blame yourself. Even if you prepare yourself, it still shreds you to pieces. I wanted him to be more normal. I wanted him to not be overcome so rapidly. I thought I could hold it at bay if I did things for him. I never let his wardrobe falter. I always had his hair combed and his nails manicured."

She talks about their move to Florida. "Four years ago he still had the cognizance to come here and check out the area. We stayed five days, and he made the decision to buy a house. I had no desire to move to Florida. It was as if I was the one with dementia. He was suddenly thinking clearly, transferring funds, and handling things like his old self. His disease was like a volleyball. One day he'd be thinking rationally, and two days later he's completely out of control. That's the real Alzheimer's.

"So he's telling his son he bought a house. His son says, 'Have the two of you lost your minds?' I said, 'Your dad was very competent through this entire transaction.' He was so proud. It was his own money."

She explains that shortly after they were married Andrew assigned power of attorney to his son to be used if he became incapacitated. "That was an agreement we spoke about before we wed. I realized that he probably wanted his children to manage his affairs, and I had no objection to that at the time. When you get married, and you're both healthy, and you both have money, you don't think that the children are going to become an issue."

She sniffs. "When we moved to Florida, they became an issue. They showed up here the second day after we arrived. We were in this empty house waiting for the furniture van. The doorbell rings, and lo and behold, it's Andrew's son and daughter. I said, 'What are you doing here?' They said, 'We came to see Dad for Father's Day.' This was the first time they ever came to see us unannounced.

"That evening when we went out to eat, they excluded Andrew completely from the conversation. There was never any real care or concern extended for their dad. They came hundreds of miles from different states to establish that their interests would be protected.

"That's the day they took him to an attorney here to have the will, trust, power of attorney, and living will drawn up. I think they felt there was an urgency because we had moved to a new state. They were concerned that new documents would have to be drawn for the state of Florida, and that perhaps their father would draw the documents to favor me more than they wanted."

She pauses, then purses her lips. "People should really be careful of durable power of attorney assignments. It's not always best for the person they're supposed to be caring for."

She explains that after this visit, Andrew's son became more and more controlling. "He was always sending me email directives. One said I was to drive Andrew to see a CPA that he'd hired in the next town. I was to have Andrew execute his tax returns, and his son would write the checks. The CPA told Andrew that he owed several thousand dollars' worth of taxes, and it thoroughly astounded my husband. He asked, 'How can I owe so much money?'

"She said there was a life insurance policy that had been cashed in, causing a tax liability of thirty-six thousand dollars. That's when I found out that his son had cancelled and cashed in the life insurance policy that I was the sole beneficiary of. I further found out that the very day that policy was cashed in, there was another policy drawn by Andrew's son and daughter as beneficiaries in the amount of seven hundred and fifty thousand dollars on Andrew's life, with an annual premium of sixteen thousand to be paid by Andrew. It was irreversible.

"When I asked Andrew how he could cancel my life insurance policy, he said, 'I trust my son, and when he puts something in front of me to sign, I sign it without questioning him.'"

The lines in Ava's face appear to deepen. "Each time he and his wife would come, they were always walking around the house pointing out which items would be for them and where they'd be placed in their house."

She gives a small shudder, then shifts gears as if she needs a break from talking about the legal issues. "We had a good social life here. We enjoyed the concerts and dining out. He would talk to everybody. As I said, when he would introduce himself, he would say, 'I'm Andrew Baldwin, and I have dementia.' The usual response was, 'We sort of have that ourselves!' It was a more comfortable setting to admit to it here.

"Then, one day he and a neighbor went to play golf. I went to get my hair done and I was running late. The men got home before I did. They drank a couple of beers on the lanai, then the neighbor went home. Andrew took a shower, put on his golf shirt, undershorts, loafers, and socks, but no pants. He walked to the cul-de-sac because he saw a Navy flag and it reminded him of his military service. He knocked on the door and told them that I had left him and wasn't coming back.

"The woman called my cell phone, but I didn't hear her with my head under the dryer. When I left the salon, I saw there was a voicemail. Her message was very tart. She said, 'How could you leave your husband by himself in the condition that he's in?' She later apologized, but that was two years ago, and after that I never left him alone.

"His condition became progressively worse. He would get up in the middle of the night and open the exterior doors, close all the interior doors, and turn all the lights on. I would awaken and say, 'Andrew, what are you doing?' He'd say, 'I'm looking for Ava.' It was like he was in another zone. I would hug him and tell him, 'I'm Ava. Everything's fine. Let's go close the doors.' That would soothe him. He'd go back to sleep immediately, and I'd be awake the rest of the night.

"It got to the point that I was run down from the lack of sleep, the stress, and his children. At times he was quite cognizant of what was going on; at other times he was oblivious. It comes and goes. You think you have a handle on it, then it regresses. As long as you're in command, you know you can face situations, but when you have other elements like Andrew's children, then you lose control. I've never been in a position where I didn't know what to do. This baffles me."

She looks across the room to the spot where Andrew's recliner used to sit.

"A letter arrived in early December. I was completely stunned to learn that his son and daughter-in-law were going to establish their residency in Florida so they could be the chief caregivers of their dad. My first thought was maybe they were going to help me out. I was having some medical issues at the time. Then I got another letter saying they were going to pick him up on a certain date. I thought, 'Andrew lives with me. This is my home! How are they going to establish residency?' Neither of them had a job, and they probably felt they could withdraw a salary out of Andrew's estate as caregivers.

"When the letters arrived, my attorney and theirs were trying to go out of town for the holidays. His son and daughter-in-law wanted Andrew, all of his belongings, and some of the furnishings. I wasn't in any condition to deal with it. I asked why they couldn't wait until January. They said they wanted him at Christmas.

"They came at nine-thirty, four days before Christmas—on the twenty-first of December—and removed Andrew first. I told him that his son was coming to pick him up. He thought he was going for a day's excursion. I fixed him an omelet for breakfast and I dressed him. Judy Simms was here when his son arrived. He left his wife outside and physically took his father. They also took Andrew's car. He asked for the keys, all the credit cards, personal effects, medical cards, and insurance cards.

"By noon they were calling a sitter because they were having such a difficult time with Andrew. They never told me that. The sitter told me. They were very much in denial. That's quite common with children."

She stops as if to catch her breath, then continues. "It was two months on the twenty-first. I haven't even spoken to him on the phone, because he can't dial. He has not been to our church since the day they picked him up. I've made five requests to see Andrew, and I've been given excuses each time. I went to see him at one of the recreation centers because I knew my neighbor would be taking him there to play pool. I went without telling his son.

"It was a complete surprise when Andrew saw me. He immediately recognized me and kissed me. He wouldn't let go of my hand. He said, 'Where did you disappear to?' and I said, 'I did not disappear. I still live at Number Two Forty-One.' He said, 'They told me you had disappeared.'

"I hardly recognized him at first. He'd lost weight. He had so much white hair on his head—like Moses—because they had not provided him a haircut. He often goes to the bathroom mirrors and speaks to himself. I can only imagine how he thinks he must look when he sees his reflection. The right side of his face from his forehead to the chin was marked from where he had been pulling and pinching at his face. He used to do that when he sundowned, but medication helped. It was quite obvious that he had not been receiving his medication.

"His daughter-in-law was constantly giving me directives of how Alzheimer's patients should be cared for. She wanted to remove his medications, because that's what they'd done for a man she once cared for. I always felt their strategies were to hasten his demise, and I feel even more so than ever that that's what they're doing. That's why I'm going to an attorney now.

"They've changed his doctors, cancelled the neurologist we used. They've taken several long trips out of state with him, which for an Alzheimer's patient is not the most favorable thing. They need structure. Even a facility would be better, because they have a routine to fit their nature. He hasn't been to a support group. They've cut him off from every friend that he had. When they found out that I saw him while playing pool, they didn't allow our neighbor to take him again for two weeks."

She blinks slowly, as if collecting her composure. "I'm handling this situation now day by day. I used to be such a strong person. I've always been focused, knowing what I had to do, which direction I had to go. Never in my seventy-three years have I felt so aimless. It's like being without a compass. I have no direction. Through people like Judy and other spiritually-minded friends, I've learned to express gratitude for so many things each morning. I'm grateful for all the friendships I have, for having this home to live in, for my own children and the support I get from my family. Before, I felt the negative forces had just overcome me, but now I'm getting my health back, and that's helping a lot. It's giving me the stability to resume some kind of life.

"I miss Andrew terribly," Ava says, her sadness palpable. "I feel he's been left without explanation. I know he's missing the touching and the hugging, the loving fellowship of his friends, and good food. Along with his mind, all of these other things have been extracted from him, and for what reason?

"There are so many lessons I've learned . . . " she slowly shakes her head. ". . . that you're really not in control of some of the situations in your life as much as you think you are. The Serenity Prayer means a lot to me. Some things you can do something about, and some things you can't."

She reaches for a glass of water, and for the first time her voice cracks. "I've also learned that when you're as low as you can get, there's going to be that divine intervention that proves itself to you. It gives you the faith to know that it's going to be all right someday, and you just have to trust and trust. I've had several of those moments by people calling, by people sending cards, and by people's hospitality and generosity."

She rises from the couch, crosses the room, and returns with a 5"x7" silver frame. Inside is a greeting card envelope with child-like scribbling in blue ink on its face. The words say, 'This is for my wife from Andreiw.' [sic]

"He did this ten months ago," she says, running her fingertips over the glass. "I got the envelope with a card I bought to send to a friend. I was annoyed at Andrew that he had taken it and written on it. Now it's one of my prized possessions."

She places the frame in her lap and pauses a moment before speaking.

"We always think our case will be different—that we will handle it, we will cope with it, and we can manage it. That's why it's important to have a good support group. We think we won't have the same problems we hear about. We deny it, we reject it, we postpone the reality, but Alzheimer's is a masterful teacher. It adjusts us to its horrors until we learn how to accept this insidious disease and deal with it. You relinquish your life—both of you do."

She shakes her head. "I don't want to show animosity, and I don't want to show anger, but Andrew and I are still legally married. He's my husband! It's the desperation of not having a game plan—of not knowing what you can do. I want to try to incorporate understanding. That's why I say that Alzheimer's is a masterful teacher. It bends you until you have no choice but to just be in it, to accept it.

"I try to keep a positive perspective. I've had enough divine intervention that I have to believe there's going to be a favorable outcome to all this. Don't ask me what that will be, because I don't know what I want."

She glances away, then softly says, "When I go to bed at night, I touch Andrew's pillow." Her eyes fill with tears and her voice is strangled. "I tell him, 'I send you love and protection wherever you are.' And I know that it's in God's hands."

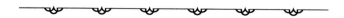

Another newcomer introduces herself to the group. A woman across the room mutters how the number of caregivers continues to grow ever higher. Eyebrows rise in agreement.

"My husband doesn't know me," the new member says, "and I'm just taking it a day at a time."

"How long has he been diagnosed?" Judy Simms asks.

"About eight months."

"Just eight months?" Even Judy cannot hide her surprise that in such a short period of time, the woman's husband doesn't know who she is.

"Yes," she says. "He went very quickly."

Another member asks, "Is he living at home?"

"Yes." She gives a weak smile.

"Well, we're glad to have you here," Judy says. "And you're going to like this group. It's very special."

Judy nods at the next member, a thin woman with burgundy hair. "Sarah?"

Sarah looks at the newcomer and speaks as if to her alone. "Being diagnosed, your heart just sinks, and your life seems to stop. But coming to this support group week after week, you get adjusted to the idea, and it's no longer an unclimbable mountain. You know you've got people behind you, and that you'll make it."

The newcomer hangs on every word. The old-timers nod in agreement.

13

VULTURES

ELAINE FORCE HAS ARRIVED EARLY for her support group meeting. She sits at a green picnic table outside the building where the meeting will be held. I join her there in the shade of a majestic oak tree draped with Spanish moss. Several ducks swim in a small pond next to our table.

As she begins to talk, it becomes apparent that Elaine's last name is ill-fitting. Rather than "*Force*-ful," today she is withdrawn and tentative. She seems to be hiding behind the large pair of dark glasses that cover her eyes. She has layered one single-colored shirt over another. Their colors reflect the way she comes across after only a few moments in her presence: black and blue.

Elaine is fifty-three years old, but she has the air of a woman who is tired beyond her years. The reason why, soon becomes apparent: Elaine is the principle caregiver for her father, who has Alzheimer's.

"My mother died four years ago from cancer," Elaine tells me. "We were so involved with her that we never saw what was going on with my dad."

I think that Elaine is referring to her father's dementia, but she is not.

"He was going back and forth to his brother's house in North Carolina," she tells me. "Come to find out, he was visiting this other woman."

The "other woman" has a family connection. She is her uncle's wife's sister—the sister of her father's brother's wife. If this seems complicated, it gets more so as Elaine explains, "Thirty years ago, my parents separated for about a year and a half. That's when my dad started seeing this woman."

We agree to call the woman Nancy.

"My mom was off doing her thing, and she decided she'd better wake up and move back into the house. My dad quit seeing Nancy, and my parents had their fifty-sixth anniversary just before she died."

Elaine takes off her sunglasses, revealing a pair of lusterless brown eyes. "My mother died in May. My dad was seventy-nine, and he kept wanting to go back to his brother's. He was going up to see this woman while my mom was sick. It was totally wrong, but my mother treated my dad like a piece of dirt, so this relationship went on. Nancy is twenty-two years younger than my father, and she's an alcoholic."

Two turkey vultures wander to within a few yards of the picnic table and peck away at the ground.

"She would travel down here to stay with him. They traveled back and forth. Then two years ago they were down here and she fell off the wagon. She got so physically sick that she couldn't eat, so my dad drove her up to North Carolina and dropped her off at the hospital ER entrance. After she got out of the hospital, she was admitted to a rehab hospital. He drove back up there a few months later and took her out of rehab against medical advice."

Elaine pulls a sheaf of papers in front of her. The pages are marked with notes and dates. She leafs through them as if looking for something in particular, then she looks up and continues her story.

"He drove her back here the next day. I kept calling his house to speak to him, and she'd answer and say, 'He's sleeping.' Finally I drove down to his house—about fifteen miles from my home—and checked his glucose. It was thirty-nine, and his blood pressure was like ninety over forty. I took him to the hospital. He had only twenty percent oxygen. Apparently, he'd been lying in the bed for three days. They did some x-rays and found out he had pneumonia so bad it engulfed the whole lung. Nancy was sitting there drunk as can be.

"So he's in the ICU, and he asked my sister and me to both come in at the same time. He told us to send her back to North Carolina, because she couldn't take care of herself. I have a brother, but he's not around much, so my sister and my daughter loaded Nancy in the car and took her directly to the hospital in North Carolina. The doctors there sent her back to the nursing home.

"It turns out my dad had given her his ATM card and password. This is where you think, 'I should be paying more attention.' She went through thousands of dollars that one week while he was in the hospital.

"One month later, after he survived the pneumonia, they diagnosed him with dementia from lack of oxygen. I think it was happening before, because one time he'd taken Nancy back to North Carolina, and they got lost for hours. They both thought it was a joke. I did ride with him, and he was pulling out in front of cars, not paying attention. That had been going on for a year or so. It got to the point where I wouldn't get in a car with him, but the lack of oxygen made it worse, so I had the doctor take away his license."

She refers to her notes again.

"Ten years earlier my dad took my brother off his Power of Attorney. He gave me the POA, but he never told my brother. I just figured they told him. When my mother died, I took care of filing all the paperwork. My husband is a funeral director and is used to advising people about those things, so we told dad we'd take care of all the legal stuff. So there we were after he was diagnosed with Alzheimer's, and I'm thinking, 'I've got the POA. I've got it under control, and everything's cool.'"

She rolls her eyes.

"So, my sister and I bought my dad a ticket to fly to North Carolina to supposedly see his brother. When he got there, he took Nancy out of the rehab hospital again, against medical advice."

She shuffles her notes, then looks at me and says with a perfectly straight face, "Pretty funny, huh?"

I tell her that it isn't funny at all.

"Come on," she says. "I can laugh." But she is not laughing.

"He broke her out. On December twenty-first he married her, which is the same day—it's the weirdest thing—my sister and I got to thinking, 'Maybe he's going to marry her.' We called the courthouse, but there was nothing anyone could do, because he hadn't been declared incompetent. He'd been diagnosed with dementia, but I hadn't been to an attorney, because I thought I had it under control."

She makes a small sputtering noise with her lips.

"So, December twenty-first they got married. They spent the next two weeks in a motel room right next to the nursing home he broke her out of. She gave him too much Viagra, and he had a stroke right there."

The sputtering is now understandable.

She runs a finger down her notes to check a date, then reports, "On January second, after my dad got back home, he told me, 'I think I had some kind of stroke.' We asked Nancy about it, and she said, 'Oh yeah. He said he didn't feel good, and was having trouble breathing.' Here we are having this conversation with her sitting in his house, and she's just like, 'Well, I don't know . . . .' Elaine shrugs to imitate Nancy's nonchalance. "She didn't call an ambulance. She didn't do anything.

"They were laughing about the Viagra. He had told me earlier that he was on eleven different drugs, and his heart doctor said not to take it. But the way his mind was, if you told him to take a pill, he'd take it.

"I took him to a doctor, and tests confirmed that he had had a stroke."

She consults her notes again. "Now we're at January of last year. I made an appointment with the family attorney who did my parents' wills. I had my brother and sister meet me there to figure out what to do about this woman, because we were afraid she was trying to kill him. My brother's wife came with him. I thought my parents had told my brother that he didn't have the POA anymore, but I guess he found out right then. He's five years older than me, and he was pretty mad.

"I'm a very quiet person," Elaine says. "His wife started yelling and screaming in front of the attorney. She accused me of stealing all of my dad's money, because on December twenty-first I went to my parents' bank after seeing what he'd done in North Carolina. I took everything out and put it in an account of my own so this woman couldn't get his money."

She returns to her stack of papers and turns a page. Finding what she is looking for, she continues.

"Starting that month, we repeatedly saw Nancy abusing my dad. She wasn't cooking for him and wouldn't let us cook for him. She gave him sleeping pills when he wasn't in pain or hurting. He wasn't eating, he couldn't swallow, and he couldn't take his medicine. That caused us to have to rush him to the ER because he was almost in a coma. She called my uncle's wife—her sister—back in North Carolina and told her that she was not going to let another ambulance take her husband away or let the hospital see him.

"I wouldn't leave him alone in the house with her, so my sister or I sat there with him, and that pissed Nancy off. She's still drinking, of course, and he's in the back of the house, sick. My sister was going through my dad's emails, and she found one from an attorney who had emailed my dad some forms to revoke my Power of Attorney. My sister called me and said, 'What's this crap?' I said, 'I don't know,' and I called the attorney. He said my dad's wife and his brother had filed to get his Power of Attorney. They wanted control of all his assets and life insurance. That's when I went to an attorney and got temporary guardianship of my father. It overrules the POA, the will, healthcare surrogate—everything," she says with a sweep of her hands, then adds, "I have a permanent one now."

Being her father's guardian did not stop the problems.

"My dad has an antique Corvette," she says, "and some guy wanted to know what time he could come by and pick it up. That's when I realized, 'Oh crap, she's trying to sell his Corvette and his other two cars!' So I got those in my name, too.

"The final straw happened when she was in the back of the house yelling at him about something. He was lying in bed and I saw her pull him up out of the bed and start shaking his head. She was standing in front of him," Elaine says, and she demonstrates by positioning her hands as if around a large melon. "She was holding his head and shaking it, saying, 'You've got to get your children out of the house! What kind of marriage is this?'"

Elaine relaxes her hands, but her face is tense. "He was very sick. He couldn't speak. He'd lost forty pounds over six to eight weeks. We got him to a hospital and found out he had a condition called *myasthenia gravis*. He pulled through it, but I don't know how he lived through that mess. They had to put a feeding tube in and feed him by liquid for three months.

"By that time, I'd called DCF—the Department of Children and Families—four times. They're supposed to protect children and elders who are being abused. I had to go to the courthouse and fill out all these papers about her abuse and what she'd done to him.

"I overheard her talking on the phone to her daughter that the two of them were taking my dad the next day to go to the bank. By then I'd moved all of my dad's money over to my account. He didn't even know it was gone. How could he not know?" Elaine asks. "I figured his dementia was still mild, but how could you not miss that kind of money?

"Then it dawned on me that it was actually my dad's aunt's money that they wanted. His aunt is a hundred and one, and at that time my father had Power of Attorney for her. You wouldn't believe the money they were taking out of her account," she says, shaking her head. "I found two withdrawals for ten thousand dollars each. I heard Nancy say, 'It's only fifty thousand. No problem. We're getting it, then we're leaving for North Carolina.'

"When I heard that, I was like, 'Oh, my God.' If there's one thing I can't stand, it's a thief. I think my dad just figured, 'It's my aunt, and she's a millionaire, so what does it matter?'" She twists her lips. "Actually, I don't know what he thought. With him and the Alzheimer's, among the three of them, they didn't have enough brains for one person.

"That's the day I went to the courthouse and had the papers done to have Nancy involuntarily committed." She explains that the DCF had advised her that invoking Florida's Marchman Act would allow her family to get Nancy into court-ordered substance abuse treatment.

"I had to go to the courthouse and fill out all these papers about her abuse and what she'd done to him. My daughter was at my dad's house, and Nancy's daughter shows up. Nancy and her daughter were trying to get my dad in the car to drive to his aunt's house to steal more money. My daughter's calling me and saying, 'I don't know what to do to keep her here!' I said, 'Call the police. I have the report here.'

"The police came, but they still could not keep the three of them from leaving the house. Somehow my daughter talked them out of leaving until I got down there with the court order to show the policeman that the sheriff's department said they would take her to a mental hospital. The sheriff showed up about seven o'clock. Nancy was drunk as a skunk. The sheriff handcuffed her and took her to the detox place. When she got out five days later, I took my dad's credit card and bought her a ticket back to North Carolina.

"After that, we had three doctors come in and deem him in-competent. That's the one thing I didn't want to do—to deem him incompetent. I thought he would hate me."

She stares at the pond and says, "I don't know if he does or not."

She speaks ever more slowly now, as if talking is an effort.

"I tried to keep my dad in his house, but running back and forth and trying to take care of him was killing me physically and mentally. I was at the point where I was ready to leave my husband. That's hard on a marriage. My husband is wonderful. He's perfect, but I was just tired. Can you imagine?

"I finally told my dad, 'It's either you or my husband.'" Her voice drifts off. "I thought my husband deserved better," she says, as she gazes at the ducks on the pond. "He's got his own bedroom now in my house. He's there all but every other weekend when my sister takes him, so my husband and I still don't have any life together. I spend every day with my dad now.

"He's very depressed. He's on very strong medicines for the *myasthenia gravis*. A therapist comes in twice a week. His muscles are sore, so he doesn't want to exercise. They bathe him twice a week, and I bathe him the other five days. I make him get up. I have him on a schedule, trying to get him more with it. He doesn't clean his own dentures. He can't shave. He can't stand for more than sixty seconds. He doesn't dress himself. I have to make sure everything's laid out, and at night I put him in his jammies, just like a baby.

"He can talk. If you ask him a question, he'll answer you, but he can't hold a conversation with you. I've asked him, 'Whatcha thinking about today?' and he'll say, 'Not much to think about.' He doesn't care about anything," she says, then gives a small snort. "Of course he doesn't. I took his wife from him."

She admits that her father's dementia is worsening. "He did get to where he wasn't wiping very good. I don't know if he doesn't care about cleaning himself. Now I have to go in there with gloves and bathe him. At least he's still going to the bathroom. I did buy diapers, because someday soon that's going to happen."

Elaine's tone is flat and emotionless as she says, "He can't do anything. He can't take his own medicine. I'll put it in front of him in the morning. I'll say, 'Here, Dad, take your pills.' Then I'll come back and he'll be sitting there staring. I try everything I can. I play games with him and cards. If he's tired of staring, he'll get back in bed, and I have to go get him out." She thinks for a moment, then says, "I would say he's in the late stages.

"The books about Alzheimer's that I've glanced through—they're depressing." She looks away, then makes eye contact. "Want the truth? I hate them. Looking at the situation now, it's like, yes, I see all that was going on with my dad, where I should have said, 'Oh, something's going on.' But I didn't, and it's depressing as heck. I feel inadequate.

"I think the hardest part is, you're mourning for this person. You remember what your father was like, and now you look at him and say, 'Where are you? Why can't you just come out for a few minutes and joke with me?' It's like I'm mourning him, and he's still there. I do still love him; it's just, he's not the same person he was all those years. He used to be fun—laughing and joking. He used to be the happy one. My mother was never happy, but he still tried to be happy."

I ask if there's anyone who can relieve some of her burden. She shrugs.

"My uncle doesn't want anything to do with him, because I stopped him from getting the POA. My brother doesn't want anything to do with me because my parents changed the POA, and I was supposed to tell him. He lives three miles from me. He calls about every eight weeks. Last year he saw him three times."

Elaine confirms that she is doing what she can to take care of herself.

"I started going to the support group. My husband met Judy Simms when he handled her husband's funeral. He told me he ran into this woman who had an Alzheimer's support group. Of course it took me months before I called her, then it took me several more months to go. I still don't like going," she admits. "The meetings are good, but I don't like talking about any of it."

She taps her notes and says, "They don't know any of this, but I thought it might help other people to see the signs, you know?" She shakes her head. "I see it in there all the time—in the group. There's another woman that comes, and her parents are both like this," she points at the papers, then adds, "and they're still driving."

"It's not that I don't care for the group," she says. "I do feel better by going, but I don't usually talk. It's great just to sit there. If I don't go, I have that guilt about not going. Isn't that weird? It's like skipping school." She shrugs. "I don't know. It makes me feel better. I don't know why. I have to figure that out . . . ."

Then, it seems as if Elaine figures it out. "I guess it's because I talk some, and I listen to them. I don't have anybody else to talk to. I mean *nobody*. Just my husband," she admits, "and he deals with families of dead people all day long. He sure doesn't want to come home and listen to me, do you think?"

The black turkey vultures waddle closer, squawking loudly.

"I can't do anything now," she says, ignoring them. "My husband and I used to travel. Now he does that with other guys. He hikes the Appalachian Trail. I used to do that with him, but I don't do that anymore. So we filed for divorce."

She notices my shocked reaction and clarifies, "Not for my husband and me! For my father and Nancy!"

We laugh together at the misunderstanding.

"I could not have filed the papers if I had not been his legal guardian," she says. "I couldn't have done anything, so I got an attorney for that, and started the divorce proceedings. We're about halfway through that process, even though Nancy is supposedly on her deathbed. The thing is, my dad could live for years, and legally she can't get any of his money now."

Elaine makes a face as if she's in on a private joke. When asked to explain, she chuckles. "We started the divorce, right? And Nancy says, 'I hate to tell you this, but your dad is the father of my thirty-year-old daughter.'" Elaine lets this bombshell land on the table, then pulls out the last page in her stack.

"In response to that, my sister came up with all this crap," she says, referring to what is on the paper. "The woman had at least four other husbands. We found the court order where she was trying to prove some other man was the father of the same daughter, and the judge threw it out."

Elaine reads aloud from the court document, "*The evidence is insufficient . . . .*"

She laughs. "I brought this so you can read it if you want." She hands across the page.

"The last paragraph is the funny part." She points to the bottom. "When the judge declared my dad incompetent, he took away all of his rights—every single one of them—except one: the right to marry."

She shakes her head, staring at the mass of papers that detail all of the problems resulting from the marriage of her mentally incompetent father. "I don't know what the heck the judge was thinking that day. 'Well, I'm going to leave him the right to marry,'" she mimics.

The turkey vultures come closer now, looking for crumbs at our feet. Elaine rests her elbow on the table and puts her head in her hand. She stares at the vultures, then says, "I think it's pretty funny."

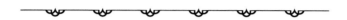

"I'm Florence, and I don't feel like talking today," the next woman says.

"That's okay," Judy replies. "We're glad you're here. Just keep coming."

Judy turns to an attractive blond woman who is next in line. "Emmy?"

"Nothing new," Emmy says. "My husband is going downhill day by day."

"How are you doing?" Judy asks.

"Well, I got the good days and bad days," she says with a slight German accent. "Last night was a horrible night, because he was up all night. He's got anxiety. Oh, that anxiety. It's almost killing him. His stomach hurts. Everything hurts, right? And when we went to the doctor not that long ago, she made him sign his name, and his signature was like a six-year-old."

Emmy turns to a younger woman beside her and introduces her daughter. "She's been here a week, and she's just doing great with him."

"Emmy has the best support from her kids," Judy tells the group.

"Oh," Emmy says, "They all come off and on, and they're really great. I was a little afraid in the beginning how they would react to him."

Her daughter nudges Emmy. "Do you want to tell the people here about the adult day care?"

"Oh! The day care! It's working! We're going there, and I drop him off and I pick him up, and he's crying all the time, but I leave him. I tell him I have to go to work in order for us to go out to dinner."

"At least, that's the story," her daughter says.

"And it works!" Emmy announces, looking quite pleased.

She then turns to Judy. "You used to say, 'You've got to lie,' and that's what I'm doing. I don't really work anymore."

Judy is quick to correct her. "We call those 'fiblets.' We don't lie."

Emmy gives her a "whatever" shrug. "I say, 'I have to go to work, Bob. We need the money,' and that keeps him from crying."

Her daughter adds, "And then when she picked him up yesterday, she said, 'Bob, I made enough money today that we can all go out to dinner,' and he went, 'Oh!'"

"See!" Judy says, "And it worked."

Emmy may be happy with the effect, but she does not seem comfortable with the cause. "It's lying, and lying, and lying."

"No, no, no, no, no!" Judy insists. "It's not lying! It's 'fiblets!'"

"I know," Emmy says, then she grins and adds, "I feel good about doing it now."

The group erupts into laughter at her impish face.

"Oh, but when you see him," she says, now shaking her head, "he's so skinny. He doesn't eat ice cream anymore. Everything he wears is loose."

"Things change," Judy says. "He'll probably find something else soon that he really likes."

"Let's hope," Emmy says with a sigh.

14

ANGST

EMMY HAHN IS SEVENTY YEARS OLD. Her short blond hair frames a sweet, round face. She wears a blue print dress and rimless glasses over gentle blue eyes. She was born in Czechoslovakia, but at age four her family left their native country as refugees and moved to Germany. She has come a long way since then, as evidenced by the small, but elegant home she occupies with her husband Bob. Oriental rugs with red tones accent dark brown leather furniture in a spotless living room. There is an afghan neatly draped over the back of one of the sofas. A young boy's likeness is incorporated into the afghan's design.

We pass through the room and take a seat at a table on an enclosed lanai. Outside, the sky is dark and threatening. An old magazine lies between us in the middle of the table. Emmy slides it toward me.

"I brought this out to show you," she says. "This is my husband on the cover." Thunder grumbles softly in the background as she adds, "This was a while back."

It is a copy of *Recycling Today*. The date on the cover is October, 1990. Bob Hahn, looking every bit the dignified executive, graces the entire page. The caption reads, "J. Robert Hahn Takes the Helm."

"He's gray now," Emmy announces, and explains that the magazine featured her husband after he opened some new factories. "We lived in Boston then. We lived in lots of places," she says with a dismissive wave.

Bob Hahn can no longer tie his own shoes, let alone run a business. He is just shy of seventy-seven, and was diagnosed with

Alzheimer's eight years ago. Today he is spending the morning in adult day care to give his wife a much-needed break.

"Before we moved here, we lived in Bonita Springs," Emmy says. "There was a doctor there who we knew well, and she brought up a word we didn't know about: 'Alzheimer's.' I don't know why she suspected, but she asked Bob some questions, and . . . ." She gives a *the-rest-is-history* shrug.

"We've been here now three years. He drove a car the first half of a year here, and one day he just gave me the keys. In the meantime, he wanted many times the key again," she says, revealing her German background with her unusual word order.

"We noticed then he had a problem. He probably had a lot more problems when we lived in Bonita, but we didn't see it. You don't want to think about it.

"There was one time the year before we came here. He couldn't put his medicine in the little boxes, and I said, 'Bob, for Christ's sake!' He said, 'Can you do that?' and I said, 'Why? What's wrong? You can't do that?'

"I gotta tell you that his mother had Alzheimer's at fifty-something. At fifty-four her husband put her into a home, but at that time, it wasn't called Alzheimer's; it was called Pick's disease. Dr. Lebron knew about it," she says, referring to Bob's neurologist. "They put his mother in this home, and she never came out. There was no medication then. Pick's disease," Emmy repeats. "I just never forgot that word."[3]

She remembers that her husband's reaction to his Alzheimer's diagnosis was anger. "He gets angry quick, but sometimes now when he gets angry . . . ." Her voice drifts off and she pulls her chin in like a turtle retreating into its shell. "He's got a temper."

---

3   According to Dr. Amanda G. Smith, M.D., Medical Director, USF Health Alzheimer's Center: Pick's disease is a separate and distinct illness that also causes progressive dementia. It predominantly affects the frontal lobes, causing early personality changes. Average age of onset is usually much earlier than Alzheimer's, and the underlying pathology (seen under the microscope) is different.

"We were sitting in Dr. Lebron's office last Friday, and Bob said something to me. I turned my head, and I saw Dr. Lebron looking at him. She saw him giving me that nasty look which is part of him. For the first time, she saw what I always see, because he usually smiles for her.

"He was taking Alprazolam for his moods. It's a little tiny pill. He used to take two or three of them a day. When she saw that look he gave me, I think it really surprised her. She told me I can give him up to five pills a day now. So when he gets a little nasty, I give him a pill, but it takes twenty minutes or so to affect him. They work, but how long they're going to work? When I took him to day care this morning, I gave the girl two pills, just in case. He doesn't like to go there. He just wants to be home with me.

"I have to put his clothes on him, because he gets confused about what he has to put on. He can't dress himself, that's for sure. That's one of the big things.

"Food, he can eat. He does pretty good. When we go out somewhere, he still uses the knife. I'm surprised he can do that. He's losing a lot of weight, though, because when we're home, all he wants to do is eat ice cream. Dr. Lebron say, 'Let him eat all the ice cream that he wants.'

"When she told me that, I said, 'Okay, I am not going to argue with him anymore. That's it.' He had very strong legs, and they're getting thinner. His stomach, with the ice cream, it's still there, but he doesn't have much of an appetite."

When asked about Bob's verbal abilities, Emmy throws out her hand. "Speaking? Oh, this is the worst. Half the time I can't understand what he is saying, so Dr. Lebron says, 'Well, go along with him.' So, whatever is in his voice, then I go with that. I play games now. That's what I'm doing. If his voice sounds like 'yes' is the right response, I say 'yes,' or if he wants me to answer 'no,' then that's what I say. If he wants me to do something, and I say yes, but then I don't do it, then he forgets about it in a few minutes. Sometimes he catches me, and he'll look at me . . . ." She mimics Bob's displeasure.

"His kids are great, though—his two sons. They do whatever they have to do. My mother died last year, and both of his boys came."

I nod toward the living room and ask Emmy about the boy whose picture is on the afghan.

"I had a daughter who died at thirty-two," she says. "She had breast cancer. Her son—my grandson—was four years old then. My daughter told him, 'Mama's going to go away, and now you're going to stay with Oma and Opa.' That's what he called us. So we adopted him. We talked about it with him first, and he said, 'I'll think about it.' He wanted our last name and the judge said, 'You're going to be a Hahn now.' So we raised him. He's twenty-five, and now he's got a little boy. He's the one on the blanket—our great grandson, Jaden.

"You know what my husband does?" she says, tilting her head. "He sits right there in that chair, and he looks at the blanket, and he talks to him. I said once, 'Does he talk to you?' and he said, 'No,' but he talks to him, and he waves. Our son was here, and he said, 'What's he doing?' I said, 'He's talking to Jaden.' So he's got serious, serious problems in his head.

"One son was visiting once, and he came running, and said, 'Emmy, give him one of those pills!' and I kind of thought, 'Good,' because he sees what's happening. Dr. Lebron says that when I can see something happening, give it to him."

Emmy gets up from the table and goes to the kitchen. She returns with a small white pill bottle. The labels reads "Alprazolam .25 mg."

"This is what he takes," she says. "He gets angry over the slightest little thing—kind of nasty. If my friend, Ava, is here, and he gets like that, she'll say, 'I think I'd better go,' and I say, 'I think so.'

"Anybody who knows Bob will know that's how he is. He was always a bit nasty, but it wasn't like this now."

I ask if she is ever worried about her safety. Emmy rocks her head from side to side.

"There was a few times, but now I won't let him get to that point. That's when I give him the medication. He'll get up in the middle of the night, and I have to follow him, and then he gets pissed off. I'm sorry to say that," she apologizes, "but that's the way it is. He can just be so angry, and he can throw something, too, but he hasn't done that in a long time.

"I learned not to argue with him. I learned to say yes or no to whatever it is. I wish I'd done that two years ago instead of going along with him, but that irritates me. It irritates me a lot when he gets angry and gets in my face. I could just shake him."

Her face is tense. Her lips form a straight, thin line.

"I used to be afraid of him, before the Alzheimer's. What I do now—and this is the truth—is I say, 'You wanna hit me? Go ahead and hit me!' and he backs up. Judy Simms says, 'You can't do that. Just let it go.' But it's hard to do.

"He was always a tough guy. He had to be, doing his work, and everything had to be his way. Now he depends only on me, and he goes along with what I say. He doesn't argue with me, as long as I'm doing the things he wants to do. I always walked a little on eggshells before, but what's different now is I take care of everything. As long as I'm with him, everything is fine, and as long as he gets those pills in him. Otherwise, I don't think I could live with him. I mean really, he just gets nasty.

"If I miss the pill, it's more constant. If he gets the pill, he's as smooth as can be." She sits back and lets her head loll to the side. "He just sits and watches a cowboy movie, although I have to give that up now because he's always talking about guns. He says, 'I'm going to get my gun out,' and stuff like that. I don't know where he got that idea with the gun. He doesn't have one, but now I can't let him watch the cowboy movies.

"In the past, when he got very angry, he had his way of getting right in your face. He never brought a knife out, but he would threaten things. He still does that. Now it scares him when I say, 'You want to hit me?' That's why he backs away. Something scares him about that."

I tell Emmy that her method sounds dangerous. She looks down, then replies softly, "I know, but I'm angry too."

She uses her chin to point at the little white bottle. "The pills are the only thing that work. I've got to give them to him. I have to make really sure that I catch him beforehand. I can tell just by words he uses or a look. That's why the doctor allows me to give him four or five a day now. That's just since last Friday. Like I said, she was writing something in his record, and when she looked up at his face, it caught her eye. The doctor tapped the table and said, 'Four of them.' I said, 'Maybe five,' and the doctor smiled just a little bit.

"So when I took him to day care this time and gave the nurse the pills, she said, 'He doesn't need it.' And I said, 'Things have changed a little bit.'

"I got all my papers done now four months ago, because who knows what happens? Some days, when he's angry, I want him out of here, but it doesn't work that way. We're all in the same boat—all of us who get together, you know? But what are you going to do?

"Going to that support group was the best thing I've ever done. It helps to understand that other people have the same problems. Judy calls me every once in a while, and she'll say, 'You call me if something goes wrong.'

"They know . . . ." She raises her eyebrows.

"Three of us couples go out after the meetings. Bob likes to go out to eat. Sometimes he gets a little irate, and he wants to go. I say, 'We can't go home. We're here with friends.' All the men have Alzheimer's. We don't go out with anybody else. I mean, you wouldn't want to do that. Nobody does. There's no conversation.

"My husband was a very big man in the business world." She points at the magazine cover. "He had plants everywhere. We lived in Italy. We went to Japan. He went to Russia—all with business. He was a very bright man, but again, his mother had it. And you know what? My mother had Alzheimer's too. She died at eighty-nine. So guess what?" She throws her hands out. "Here I am. We'll see. What're you gonna do?

"I do feel sorry for him. Do you know how bad it is when you've been a man like this, and then you're nothing? Last year he wet the bed a lot. He hasn't done that in a while. I keep the light on so he can find his way to the bathroom, but then he'll go in the shower. That's why I hear everything.

"I have to watch him all the time. He goes from room to room opening cabinets, and he brings stuff out. This is something brand new the past weeks. Many times I can't find something I'm looking for, so now I hide my purse.

"I was only in Germany three or four times a year with my mother, but the real Alzheimer's is right here in the house with my husband, day to day. You wake up in the morning, and you're not sure what he's going to be like today. Is he going to be in a bad mood? Am I going to do something to make him angry? Because you know," she purses her lips, "I'm not perfect. I get angry a lot over him. I could belt him," says sweet Emmy Hahn. "Yes, I could, but I wouldn't get very far, I don't think.

"You just go from day to day, hour to hour. When I pick him up from day care, sometimes he's angry, and sometimes he says, 'Where've you been?' and there are tears in his eyes. I say, 'I told you, I'm working at Beall's department store.' And I'm really not, but I tell him, 'I'm working so we can go out to eat.' He says, 'We have money,' and I say, 'Not so much anymore,' which isn't true. He doesn't say, 'Well, we don't have to eat then.'

"People are laughing at the support group meetings. Somebody reminded me the other day after I said I was going to go and do something, 'Well, you're working at Beall's, aren't you?'

"You know, I'm a nervous wreck by the time I get to the day care to pick him up, because you never know what's coming out of him. That's why I told the girl, 'Give him the second pill before I get there.' I give him a little note that says, 'I'll be back at two-thirty,' and he reads the note the whole time he's there. I get in the car, and then I drive home, like this morning, and I know I have a few hours to myself.

"One day I did nothing but watch old movies. I could just sit here. I forget things for a while, then I'm a nervous wreck again when I go to pick him up. I don't know. It's just hard. But I am very happy that all the kids are coming a lot."

Emmy shares her regret that her neighbor moved away. "Her husband had Alzheimer's, too, so she was wonderful with Bob. Once, about a year ago, we must have had an argument. He went over there, and he was going to stay there. She got him to calm down, but I went over and said to him, 'What the heck are you doing?' She said, 'You gotta say yes, if that's what he wants to hear.'

"We didn't have him on any medication then. He started with the Aricept—the one in the bottle—but I don't think it worked with him. That's when you could give it to him and he still would be angry. That's when we changed it to the patch." She leaves the room and returns with a sample patch.

"It's called Exelon Patch 9.5 mg.," she says, handing it across the table. "He wears it on his back, or chest, or arm every day. Everybody's hoping they're going to bring something better out, but so far, nothing's happening. You can tell sometimes when it wears down, or if it comes off when he showers, or if he scratches himself. One time he came out and it must have fallen down, because a few hours later he was different.

"I thought to myself, 'Did I put the patch on?' and it was off. So then it takes a little while again to kick in. He'll get kind of ticked off about something, some slight thing. If he wants something and we don't have it, he gets agitated. That's why I listen to every little word now. Good thing Dr. Lebron says, "Give him whatever he wants,' like the ice cream." Emmy shudders. "Oh God, yeah. I always have a lot of ice cream here. I've got it in the garage and in the kitchen."

If she could turn back the clock, Emmy admits that she would accept his condition right from the start.

"I didn't do that. And I wouldn't argue with him." She slaps the table. "Oh, God, I've been in so much trouble because I argue with him. My neighbor says, 'Don't argue with him. Just say yes.' I ask her, 'How do you do it?' and she says, 'I've learned through the years.'

"I say, 'I can't do this. He's irritating me. I want to call him every name,' and she says, 'Don't do it.' Sometimes I still speak out, and I'm like this . . . ." She clenches her fists. "Then, afterwards, I think, 'Stupid me!'"

She relaxes her hands and flops back in her chair. "I don't know. I wish they'd come up with some medication. Something big."

She glances into the living room at the afghan, then says, "You know, we have sometimes some good times, and then you forget about it for a little while. That's when I forget to give him a little pill, then I have to be really nice for half an hour until it starts working. He's got this anxiety that's driving him crazy, I think. He expresses it by being nasty and taking it out on me. I don't get a lot of sleep. He's got a problem with sleeping. He's got this anxiety that keeps him awake, so I bought some sleeping things from Walgreens. Then I give him another of those little pills, and then I get at least five hours sleep."

I ask Emmy what she does to let off steam.

"My best stress reliever is when he's not here. What else can there be? That is the best. I will not pick him up until two-thirty. I could leave him there until five o'clock, but then I feel guilty that I leave him there too long. You wouldn't believe what it's like when I drive him there." She rolls her eyes. "Oh, boy. Most of the time he doesn't know where we're going, then one time we got there and he said, 'I'm not going in there.' For just a minute the darkness went away, and he knew what was going on. Those shadows move, and they can lighten up. Sometimes I hear him say things, and I think, 'Where did that come from?' and then ten minutes later, it's gone. One minute he can be so friendly and nice, and then the next minute he's as nasty as can be.

"So I go walking around the lake. I would do something different, but where the heck can you go? We were told a long time ago by Dr. Lebron that he cannot go to a different place. She said, 'You cannot travel with him.' We went to Virginia last year to visit my son, and it was a nightmare. Bob wasn't home in his own bed. He panicked in the security line at the airport, because they wouldn't let me go through with him. This was last year when he wasn't even that bad. The doctor said, 'I told you, you cannot travel with that man anymore.'

"When he panicked, I tried to tell those people, 'Leave him here by me; he's got Alzheimer's,' but they didn't seem to understand that, because they follow their rules. This is something they should know about—this Alzheimer's."

She agrees this would have been a good time to hand out the small blue cards that say, "My partner has Alzheimer's. Thank you for understanding."

In the meantime, Emmy admits, "I'm walking on eggshells, and everybody at the meetings knows about it. It's so wonderful to go there and let it out. Besides, I get rid of him for a while when I go there. I think he likes it down the hall in the respite care room. He's got friends there. They talk and talk, and they don't know what they're talking about, but at least they're talking. Now, if I talk with somebody, Bob gets angry, because he thinks I'm talking about him—and he's right."

Emmy sighs. "When the ending is of all this, I don't know. It's up to Dr. Lebron when the time comes to put him in a home. She just says, 'It's not time yet.' I understand this, because I can still handle him, but is it going to be six months from now? What does he have to be like before we could put him in a home? I'm just going to hold on and see what happens."

As she speaks, a bolt of lightning flashes across the dark sky. It is followed almost instantly by a crash of thunder. Rain begins to splatter against the lanai windows.

Emmy glances at the black clouds, then admits, "I'm afraid sometimes—a little bit—of what it's going to be like ahead. Dr. Lebron said, 'Your day will come.' She didn't look at me when she said it, but she must have said that to me, and not to Bob. It was like, 'Just hang in there.'

"That's how I look at it," she says, with a sigh. "So, I'm just hanging in there, and I'm going to keep him at home as long as I can."[4]

---

4   One month after this interview with Emmy Hahn, Bob Hahn became ill and was admitted to a local hospital. After a three-day stay, he was transferred for the long-term to a bed at Arbor Village nursing home. Reports from Emmy Hahn's support group reveal that Emmy is like a new person.

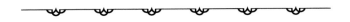

Judy turns to a woman with medium length red hair and wire-rimmed glasses. "Okay, Linda . . . ."

"My husband has been at Arbor Village for almost three months, and it's a constant, 'When am I going to go home? How long am I down for?' which is a prison term," Linda says with a laugh, "because he used to be a prison guard. I tell him he's here for rehab. He said one day, 'If you want to put me in a home, just go ahead. I'll survive.'

"At first he thought this was a vacation. He'd say, 'I don't know why we came here. This really isn't a very nice place. The food's pretty good, and the waitresses are really nice, but next time, let's not come here.'"

The group laughs.

"Even the other day he said that, but they're going to let him come home two weeks from today."

Judy's eyes grow wide and she utters an ominous, "Ohhh . . . ."

"So he knows he's going home," Linda says, "but he'll say, 'Now, where are we going?' and I have to give him the address. I can't just say 'home' because he really isn't sure where that is. The other day he couldn't find something. They changed his room, and that's so confusing for them. So, I'm concerned. They think I can manage. They said in sixty-six days, if I can't manage, and if he gets worse, I can bring him back."

Judy looks concerned as well.

"Another thing you should know about," Linda says, "is that I've filled out the Medicaid information. I even got the financial people you all recommended to help me with that, but I'd still have to pay twenty-four hundred dollars

a month, which is more than half of our income. I don't know how I'm supposed to do that."

Around the table, heads nod up and down.

Linda crosses her arms. "I go from being glad he's here, to wishing he was home, to wishing he would just drop dead."

Not a soul in the room looks shocked.

"Just hang in there," Judy says.

"I know that sounds horrible," Linda says, "but there are days when he can be so mean to me. When he gets really hateful for no reason, you go from one extreme to the other, which is very tiring."

She blows a burst of air through her lips. "I got two more weeks. Then we'll see."

15

You Have to Laugh

LINDA SPITLER INVITES ME INTO THE MODULAR HOME that she shares with her husband, John. We take a seat in the living room on matching striped couches. John is home, but there is no sign of him. It's one o'clock, and Linda explains that he is in bed.

"There's nothing else for him to do," Linda says with a thick Virginia accent. "He can't follow a plot on TV, and he eats too much. He sleeps all the time, and whenever he gets up he wants to eat. Yesterday he got up at eleven o'clock and had something to eat. So at twelve-thirty he wanted lunch. I said, 'But you ate a whole meal an hour and a half ago!' and he said, 'It's twelve-thirty, and it's time for lunch, and I'm still getting another meal today!' He always thinks I'm trying to talk him out of a meal.

"So I fixed him something to eat, and he said, 'How many people do you serve every day?' I said, 'Just you and me,' and he said, "Then how do we make any money?'"

She rolls her eyes, but there's a slight smile in those eyes.

"He was diagnosed about four years ago, but looking back, I can see things weren't right for probably the last ten. So, he's further along than you would think. Every morning he says 'I'm dying. I'm probably going to die today,' and I say, 'Well, not today.'"

John is seventy-three and Linda is sixty-six. They have been married for twenty-seven years. "On our twenty-fifth anniversary, we re-did our wedding vows, because I thought it was important. 'For better or worse,' and 'in sickness and in health' doesn't mean much when everybody's healthy," she says. "It means a whole lot when things change.

"He knows that he's not right. He doesn't really know what this dementia is, but he'll ask me, 'How long does it last? What can you do for it? When are you going to take me away?' I've told him in more lucid times that that may happen, but today we just worry about today.' He was in the military for twenty-five years, and he was a police officer, and then he was a prison guard, so he's not used to not being in control.

"He says, 'I don't know why you don't just shoot me.' Last week he said it again, and I told him, 'Well, I can't do that.' And he said, 'Yes, you could. You're just concerned about yourself, and that's just selfish! I'll write you a note, and they'll know it's okay if you shoot me.'"

She tells all of this with a half-smile. I ask if there are guns in the house.

"There are, but there aren't any bullets. He still asks about his guns once in a while. I don't think he would commit suicide, but he wants to be dead, so if somebody else would do it, that would be fine with him.

"The other day I was explaining to him that I was filling out the forms for the brain bank so the researchers will learn something from his brain, and he said, 'Okay, I'll do that. Tell them to come and get it.' I said, 'That's after you die!' and he said, 'I thought they could just put me to sleep and take it.'

"One time he asked the doctor, 'Why can't you just give me a shot and put me to sleep?'

"He says things like that a lot, and if I speak to him in a joking way, it's okay, so I told him, 'You have to go to the veterinarian for that.'" She gives a wry smile.

"Six months ago he fell and couldn't get up, so I had to call an ambulance. They took him to the hospital for three days, and then they took him to the nursing home. You have to be hospitalized for three days, then Medicare will pay for one hundred days in a home. After his hundred days were up, they told me he qualified to stay because he was bad enough. The thing is, because he could feed himself, dress himself, and get from the wheelchair to the bed and toilet, if I wanted to take him home I could.

"Every day he asked, 'When can I come home?' The guilt was awful. Everybody will tell you that. So I brought him home." She looks around her. "He doesn't know this house. We've lived here eleven years, and he doesn't know where the bathroom is. He still asks me, 'When can I go home?' So I ask him, 'Where is it you want to go?' He says, 'I don't know, unless it's Heaven.'

"He has no memory of being in the nursing home, so if he has to go back, I hope I won't feel that guilty again. They told me I was lucky he got in there, and I should leave well enough alone and leave him there. Now I have to wait for him to fall again and go back to the hospital so that Medicare will pay for it.

"I was shocked when they told me that when our time ran out we were going to have to pay $2,487 dollars a month to keep him there. That's better than half of our monthly income. I worked in a garment factory for thirty years. My pension for thirty years is ninety-four dollars a month. My Social Security is eight hundred dollars a month. They'll take most of his. Wouldn't you go 'Aagh!' if your monthly income was going to be cut in half?" she asks as her fingers curl into claws.

"So I'm trying to keep him home long enough to come up with a way to get twenty-five hundred a month. I may have to go find a job. I get really frustrated with the Veterans' Administration. The man gave twenty-five years of his life to the Army. A lot of the veterans' hospitals are not set up for dementia patients. There's a veterans' place a little ways away that takes patients, but the price isn't going to be any better than here, where he's five miles away.

"So I don't know what I'm going to do." She picks up a glass of iced tea and takes a slow sip. Her frustration is palpable.

"Right now it's one day at a time. I don't think he needs to be in the home as much as I need him to be in there. I'm gaining weight because I can't get out and exercise. I'm just sitting here getting fatter and lazier. I have friends that stay with him while I go to the support group, but if I go to the grocery store or go to get a haircut, it's hard to make an appointment because I don't know how he'll be at that time. This morning I went to Bible study and I felt guilty. I just put him to bed and said, 'Stay here and I'll be home.' I'm lucky he can sleep.

"Someday I'll find he's fallen, and that'll be the end of that. He stopped smoking because he won't walk as far as the porch to smoke. He doesn't wander. Instead, he calls me a lot and says, 'What're you doing?' He has no opinions, because he can't follow anything. People don't come to visit, because he can't hold a conversation. He doesn't know who they are half the time. Then there's the folks that say, 'Well, we could stop by, but we don't want to see him like that.'" She rolls her eyes.

The picture she paints is bleak, and her voice chokes as she admits, "My life has changed so much. Sometimes I resent it, and then I feel guilty, because it's not his fault.

"My mother passed away not long ago, and we had a funeral here," Linda says, crying now, "but her family is in West Virginia. We're planning on a memorial service and a family reunion there, and I really don't want to miss that, but we're not going to be able to go. Our church is just five miles away, and just to drive between here and there the other day, he asked me six times, 'Where are we going?' and 'How much longer?' I could not take thirteen hours of that.

"He gets confused here, asking, 'Where's the bedroom?' and 'Where's the bathroom?' You take him in a hotel, and it could be a horrendous night. I don't know if I could take him in a restaurant. I know I couldn't take him in a rest area bathroom. An airport would be just as bad." She shudders at the thought.

"A friend of mine brought her husband down here. He has Alzheimer's too, and he got really bad because of the traveling." She jerks a thumb toward the kitchen and says, "He was so confused that he was peeing in the refrigerator, so they flew him back, but he kept trying to pull back the curtain to First Class. It was The Trip from Hell. So, you think, 'Okay, we'll just stay here' but I'm not going to miss my mother's memorial service, so I guess I'm going to have to find some place that he can stay for a couple of weeks while I'm gone."

Suddenly, from the back, a man yells out, "Can I pee?"

"Yeah!" Linda yells back.

"That's mighty nice of you," John Spitler responds.

"He always has a little bit of a sarcastic, smart-ass mouth," Linda says, "considering the people he's dealt with over the years."

John's voice grows louder now, and his words paint a picture of his condition that is more clear than anything Linda has said to this point.

"Jibber-jabber!" he says loudly. "If you say so!" he adds, even though no one has said a word. "Jibber-jabber!" he says again, then shouts, "Where do you want me, Linda?"

"Come here and talk to the lady, and you can have ice cream," she answers.

"Oh, wow," he drawls with what sounds like sarcasm.

"I'm having to come up with treats all the time now, because he gets bored," she explains as she gets to her feet. "I'll go bring him out."

She disappears down a hallway. I hear her explaining to John that I am writing a book about Alzheimer's. The thumping of a cane announces his arrival.

"He couldn't get the hang of a walker," Linda says as she emerges from the back with her husband. John is tall and imposing, standing well over six feet. He wears a pair of glasses on his bristly face. His head is bald on top, with close-cropped gray hair on the sides. He is wearing slippers, pajama bottoms, and a white t-shirt.

"Where do you want me?" he asks, stopping at the entrance to the living room.

"Come over here and sit in mother's chair," Linda says as she guides him toward a kitchen chair that she has placed between the two sofas.

"Where?" he shouts in an abnormally loud voice.

"Right here."

"Boo!" he says, looking at me, then laughs.

I introduce myself, and he replies, "This is John, who's getting ready to fall. Did you write that down?"

I tell him that I'm writing everything down, if that's okay with him.

"Oh, my God," he says with wide eyes.

"Are you having me sit down into nothing?" he asks Linda behind him.

"No, there's a chair here."

She gets him settled, then returns to her seat on the couch. We have not discussed how this part of the conversation will go, but with no prompting from me, Linda begins to interview her husband.

"Are you aware of what's going on with you," she asks, "that you have Alzheimer's?"

"Oh yes, aware," he says. "Oh yes."

"How has it changed your life?"

He screws up his face. "How has it changed my life? My thinking. The way I react to certain things. I'm not capable of doing a lot of things I used to be able to do . . . understanding things."

His answer is surprisingly coherent after his previous outbursts.

"His neurologist says he's bad," Linda says, as if reading my mind, "but he's good enough to know how bad he is."

I ask if he's making an extra effort because of my visit.

"He's very good right now," she answers, "and a lot of times he is, but tomorrow he won't remember you. He won't know about the book. I'll have to tell him every time I mention the book."

"Well, you lost me already," John says. "What's the book?"

"See?" says Linda.

John twirls his index finger in a circle by his ear and whistles, as if to say, "*The guy is looney-tunes . . . .*"

"Is it frustrating to you?" Linda asks.

He twists his mouth again as he thinks. "It's frustrating, yes. You just gotta live with it. It takes a while for you to understand that you're not the way you used to be, and that you're not able to do certain things you used to do."

Linda takes advantage of this opportunity to ask, "When you get up every morning you tell me you're going to die today. Do you really feel that way?"

"Oh, I'd give anything to die," he says. "That would be the best gift anybody could give me right now. Let me pass away nice, quiet, and peacefully . . . no harm to anybody."

Linda's face shows no emotion.

"What are you looking forward to every day?" she asks.

"There's nothing to look forward to, Linda," he says flat out. "There's just nothing. I get up and I eat." He shrugs his shoulders. "I'm not upset. I just know that there's not that much to look forward to that day. I'm going to eat and try to keep my mind busy, but I'm just . . . . I don't know how to explain it to you. What am I here for? I have no ambition. There's nothing I gotta do. There's nothing I can get done. I'm just here."

"If I told you right now to drive to town, could you do it?" she asks.

He thinks for a moment, then answers, "Yeah, I guess I could."

"Would you know where the car keys are?" she asks, "and where to turn?"

"I think I could get there," he says. "It might be a real quick trip."

"Do you remember being at Arbor Village?" she asks about the time he spent in the nursing home.

"I know the name Arbor Village."

"But you don't remember being there for a hundred days."

"There are a lot of things I don't remember."

"Why do you tell me to throw you away?"

"Because I'm a waste," John answers. "I'm not doing anything. I don't think that's hard to understand."

"Are there things that still bring you happiness?" she asks, as if she has a script.

"Oh . . . ." He pauses. "Things like kinfolks coming in."

Linda makes a face that clearly says, "When's the last time anyone came to visit?"

She turns to me now and says, "When the diagnosis came in, I already knew."

"Oh, you did?" he says to her. "I knew I had something, but I didn't know what it was."

"It's one thing to see it coming," she says, "but then down the road the doctor's saying, 'We need to get him on medication,' and it's like, 'Oh, crap, it's really here.'"

"I told some of his family about it, because both of his parents had dementia," she says to me.

"Both of mine did?" John asks.

"Yeah. I told them it scares me to death."

"Amazing," John says. "I don't remember all this."

"In the last two years, things have really gone downhill."

"And I missed 'em!" he laughs.

Linda seems to have finished interviewing John, so I ask her to describe the *real Alzheimer's*.

She stares at her husband as she answers. "It's the frustration of not being able to do what we planned to do when we moved down here. It's the things I can't do, even though it's not me who's sick. That makes me angry, then you have the guilt that comes from something that's nobody's fault. I feel more like a mother than a wife. I feel like a short-order cook lately. It's just . . . ." she struggles to find the words, then thinks of an example:

"Somebody brought their daughter to one of the support group meetings. The caregivers were hard on her, telling her, 'You don't understand.' She finally said, 'I guess in a way you're right, because my life hasn't been disrupted.'

"My life has been disrupted!" Linda says, as more of her frustration bubbles to the surface. "It has been disrupted socially, financially, sexually . . . . Every aspect of my life has been changed, and it will always be changed. When this is over, it will be changed again. For that daughter who came to the meeting, she goes back to her life, and when her mother is gone, she'll go back to her life. Everything about our life is changed. We can't go on vacation, we don't go out to eat, we don't go to parties, we have to watch the money very carefully . . . ."

John has been listening quietly, and now he says, "We do some of those things."

"So how has your life changed?" she asks him.

"I didn't know it had changed that much until you started talking," he says, making a silly face.

"That's why you're lucky to have me," she cracks back. "Everything's good for you, right?"

"No. Everything's not good," he says, "but I didn't know it was that bad! You're supposed to cheer me up."

"We need to tell her the truth," Linda says, nodding at me.

"And the truth will set you free!" he says in a loud sing-songy voice.

She ignores this outburst and says to me, "He frustrates me, and I frustrate him, but I don't always know what he wants from me, and I don't always give him what he wants. Sometimes we'll snap at each other, and we're both immediately sorry. We do love each other very much, and we don't hesitate to tell each other that."

They look into each other's eyes. John is quiet.

Linda turns to me. "The only way you can take this is one day at a time, because every day's different. It's up and down, and you know there's no way out. There's no light at the end of the tunnel. This won't end until he passes away, so that's not a light. To say that's the only thing I have to look forward to is too depressing, so you don't think too far ahead.

"Financially I have to think ahead. Physically I have to think ahead—like where I'm going to end up—but you don't know until the time comes. So, mostly you can't plan. I can't even plan a haircut."

"A lot of times I just wish I'd go ahead and croak," John says, "but that's up to the good Lord."

Linda makes no reaction to his comment. Instead, she says, "Everybody at the support group knows exactly how I feel, and I know how they feel. We need to talk about things, and we all listen. There are people there whose husbands haven't even been diagnosed yet, but they're there because they think something's wrong. They sit and listen to this lady who's having to deal with a feeding tube for her husband, so the whole thing is laid out from end to end. I'm somewhere in the middle.

"I've only missed one meeting since I started going when he first went in the nursing home. He was diagnosed several years ago, but I thought, 'Why do I need to go talk to people that have the same problems I do?' But there's information there that I couldn't have known, like about the financial services. There's a lot of emotional support, too.

"This one woman's husband just passed away. He was violent and smart-assed for a long time, and she was crying and said, 'I can't get over all the times I told him I wished he'd just drop dead!' Occasionally that thought crosses your mind, and who can you say that to, except people who understand how you feel?

"Sometimes with him," she says, nodding at John, "sometimes he's back there in bed and it's like having a child. Sometimes I wish he'd get up so I could play with him, and then he gets up, and I wish he'd go back to bed."

Hearing this, John fakes crying like a baby. His wails are inappropriately loud.

"But I enjoy the support group," she says, ignoring his theatrics. "I have friends that come here every Monday so I can go to the group without paying for home care. That's who your real friends are, not the ones who say, 'If you need anything, call me.' It's the ones who just come."

I ask Linda if she wishes she'd gone to the support group earlier.

"It would have helped," she admits, "but I didn't really think I needed it. You think, 'What's the big deal? I can handle it myself.' Most people are surprised after they go how much it helps. I was surprised, and now I look forward to it every week, even if I don't have anything to say. It helps just to sit with people who know what it's like.

"The first two months I went, I would cry at every meeting, and nobody minded. They kind of expected it, and it was okay. You cry in front of other people who aren't going through this, and they're like, 'Put your big girl pants on and buck up; it's not so bad!' But there, you can cry and fuss and it's okay. I think we need a lot more support groups. There are three people within walking distance of my house with the same problems, so it would be nice if we could have a meeting in here. I don't know if I have the strength right now, but maybe someday. . . . ."

I ask if they have any advice for other couples who are facing what they're going through.

"You have to keep your sense of humor," Linda says. "If we didn't laugh at some of the stuff that happens . . . ." Her voice drifts off and she shakes her head. "That's what keeps us going. We've always had a lot of fun."

"Yup," John agrees.

"He's incontinent now," Linda says, "and every morning I have to change the sheets. Sometimes I even have to change the blankets and the spread, and he'll say, 'Boy, I really sweat.'

"The other day when I was changing the sheets again, he asked me, 'Whose house is this?' I said, 'It's our house.' He said, 'How did it get to be our house?' and I said, 'We bought it,' and he asked me, 'Why did we buy a house with piss all over it?'"

John smiles, but it's not clear if he knows why Linda is laughing.

"We both have a sense of humor," she says.

John looks at me now and announces, "You've got six toes on one foot." He pauses while I look at him, trying to figure out where this is going, then he says, "You never counted them?"

I glance down at my feet, and John laughs heartily, pleased that he has demonstrated his sense of humor.

"You have to accept it," John says, and I know that he is lucid enough now to be speaking about Alzheimer's and not my toes.

"You know something's there," he continues, "and you have to get used to understanding what you can and can't do about it. You have to learn to live with it, and that's not easy."

Linda jumps in again. "He said this morning, 'When are you going to throw me away? When are you going to put me somewhere? Why do you put up with this?' Sometimes, if I'm having to dress him or change him—especially if he has a 'number two' accident, which doesn't happen too often—I want to pop my rubber gloves at him and say, 'I'm going to get you.'" She mimics pulling back a slingshot.

"The other day I was cleaning him up after another accident, and it was really a mess. When I was all done, I said to him, 'Come on. Let's go in the kitchen and I'll make you breakfast,' and he said to me, 'Are you sure you want to feed me again?'"

John beams, and Linda says, "Then one day he told me, 'I pray for you every day,' and I thought, 'Well, now, how about that—for him to pray for me?'

"But I told him that his disease is not something that's going to go away. His mother had it, and I told him that's where he's going. I told him, 'It breaks my heart to see you like this, and I know there's no cure, so all I can do is pray you go soon and without a lot of pain.' Then I told him, 'When you get to Heaven, pick us out a really nice house with a lot of windows,' and he said, 'Okay.'

"So, you know, I have no problem with letting him go. I get kind of excited about going to Heaven, so why do I dread him going? Now, when the time comes, that might be different . . . .'" Her voice drifts off.

"I had some chest pains a few weeks ago," she says, "and I thought that maybe I should go in for a stress test, but then, who would look after him? If they told me I need a catheter test, that would take a whole day, and who would watch him? So I just thought, I can't do that right now, which is part of the reason they say the caregivers die before the one that has the disease. We had one of the guys who comes to our meetings die of a heart attack a few weeks ago."

"Can I get some food here?" John asks out of the blue.

Linda glances at him, then tells me, "The other day I was making lunch and he asked me, 'Who runs this place?' I told him, 'I guess I do.' He asked me, 'Am I the only patient?' and I said, 'Yes, thank God.' Then he asked me, 'Who does this place belong to?' and I said, 'It's our house. We bought it.' He asked, 'Do we own it?' and I said, 'We make payments on it.' So he asks, 'How much are the payments?' and when I told him, he said, 'How do we make any money, if I'm the only customer?'"

We both smile at John, who squints, then scratches his head.

"See what I mean?" Linda says, "A sense of humor helps."

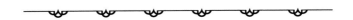

"Okay," Judy smiles at a man who has been sitting quietly in the corner. "Mr. Bob?"

The man looks as if he wishes Judy would have passed him by. His Adam's apple moves up and down, he blinks, then he speaks.

"Well, things are going about the same. My wife Jean lives at home. She was diagnosed two years ago. Of the seven stages on the Alzheimer's website, I estimate she's about stage four. She still takes care of herself, but I have to remind her about her pills. She can't do any emails, and she can't do the checkbook. I have to supervise her cooking to make sure she doesn't over-season or burn things.

"Last week we went down and saw her cousin. There was a group of people there, and I said, 'I know that guy over there. He's the guy that does the Geico commercials.'" Bob imitates the familiar deep voice, and everyone laughs.

One woman asks, "Does he really talk like that?"

"Yeah, he does," Bob says, adding, "and I got to meet him, so that's pretty much it."

Judy squints at him. She purses her lips, then says, "You're not going to tell us how you feel?"

"How I feel?" Bob asks.

"Yes," she says. "How you're <u>doing</u>."

"I'm trying to cope," Bob says, with a hint of defensiveness.

A woman across the room asks, "Are you succeeding?"

"Well," he says, "in the dilemma with Jean's daughter, yes. She sends me this four-page letter about how frustrated she is, trying to talk to me. I can't compete with her verbally, so I just send simple statements back. So that's kind of the way it's going."

"Do you have your paperwork done?" Judy asks. "Your Power of Attorney?"

He flashes a quick smile, and nods. "We have the Power of Attorney, the will, and the health care surrogate, and we did go to the bank to find out about some other financial things. We changed all of the beneficiaries to her daughter, so in case Jean does get placed, we've got all that. She's also signed up for the brain bank."

"That's good," Judy says. "Anything else?"

"Nope," Bob says. "That's it."

Judy moves on to the woman sitting to Bob's right. The woman asks if anyone knows about a list of "The Ten Absolutes for Caregivers."

"It has all those things you should or shouldn't say to someone with Alzheimer's," she says.

Another woman raises her hand and comments, "That list can turn a whole day around for you."

Judy knows about the list. She has seen it printed on laminated pieces of paper the size of business cards. "Does anybody have one?" she asks.

Bob speaks up. "I made those."

The woman on his left asks, "You wrote the list?"

He shakes his head. "I found it somewhere and made up those cards."

"That means so much," the woman says.

Bob smiles shyly and says, "I'll make some more."

16

FEELINGS

BOB JAMESON IS PROUD OF HIS TIME IN THE MILITARY. His blue ball cap shows "U.S. Navy Veteran" in gold lettering above the brim. It is warm at the picnic table where we sit, but in addition to his ball cap, Bob wears a tan *Members Only* jacket. When I comment on the Navy insignia, he gives a quick grin, then pulls the jacket back to reveal a Navy logo on his light blue polo shirt as well.

Bob is seventy years old. His wife Jean is seventy-four and was diagnosed with dementia two years earlier, but her illness is not the only thing on Bob's mind.

"My veteran's group has taken a big hit lately," Bob says. "Seven members of our local chapter have died in the last six months."

He raises his eyebrows and leaves this stunning statistic hanging in the humid air before stating, "My mother passed away eighteen months ago. I went through six years of her having dementia from a stroke, and that's the reason I was able to pick up on my wife's problem so quickly.

"Jean and I have been together for twenty-five years and married for twenty-one. About three years ago we were in our travel trailer, and she couldn't remember things. There was no real 'aha' moment. It was just an accumulation of things.

"I told her, 'I'm beginning to worry that something's wrong with you.' About a year after that, some of the neighbors started noticing there was something different, too. I got her to the doctor, and she took a big battery of tests."

He picks up a large manila folder that has been lying at his side and pulls out a sheaf of papers. "This was the initial report," he says, handing across the first page.

The report notes Jean's cognitive decline and states that her testing was most consistent with a vascular dementia, but that they could not rule out the possibility of a confounding Alzheimer's disease.

Bob hands across a second page and says, "And this was the follow-up."

The report's summary states, "The results of today's neurocognitive evaluation are of concern . . . We are additionally concerned that she exhibits a degree of confusion that is not typical of a vascular dementia profile (pointing to Alzheimer's)." In addition to medication, the doctors recommended that Mrs. Jameson discontinue driving.

"Jean didn't like the part that said she couldn't drive anymore," Bob reports. "She lost her independence, and in a way, I lost some of mine, too, because now anytime she wants to go somewhere, I have to take her. She always had a problem finding her way someplace, but that was just normal. What they were concerned with was if she got into a situation and had to make a quick decision, she'd be like this:" He holds up both hands and makes a frantic face.

"There was one lady in the support group whose husband was using cruise control going down the highway, and he forgot how to turn it off. He was driving a lot longer than he should have." Bob shakes his head. "I've seen some scary ones . . . ."

He puts the doctor's report back in his folder and says, "When I read the results, I actually thought it wasn't that bad. At that point, one of my biggest fears was going broke. When I went through it with my mother, we had to sell her property and use up all her money so she could go on Medicaid. I didn't know about being married and being able to get on Medicaid without losing everything.

"It wasn't until I started with the support group a little over a year ago that I found out I might not ever be rich, but I wasn't going to go broke. Brenda Lee Ray came to our house, and she took a big load off of me just by telling me that."

With his financial concerns alleviated, Bob is now learning to cope with the gradual loss of his wife's abilities.

"There's a new problem every week. She can't put her pills out anymore. I have to sort them, and remind her to take them. The week before last she put her shoes on the wrong feet. She can't write checks anymore. Right now I have to write the checks and then she'll sign them. She has to practice writing her name first. She still does the dishes, she showers, and she gets dressed. It takes her forever, but . . . ." He looks away as he states, "It's just a very slow, progressive thing."

Bob tells how he and Jean used to go to Alzheimer's support group meetings for his mother. "I went to the group where she lived just to find out what this was all about," he says. "A lot of the people there were in a lot worse shape, because they'd tried to take care of their spouses for ten or fifteen years. They were just like this one woman in the group I go to now." He holds his arms out to the side and shakes like a person having a seizure, saying, "She's still got her husband at home, and she's a nervous wreck.

"I started going to the support group meetings here a year ago January. There was a newspaper ad about them. I looked and I found it, and it helps being with other people that understand. Average people don't understand, and they either don't want to be bothered, or they run away from it. You lose your friends. They start avoiding you.

"I'm the token male in the meetings sometimes," he says with a laugh. "I guess maybe I'm not as macho as some men who might refuse to come. There are about three of us regulars. We had one more, but he passed away recently."

He flashes a quick smile. "I listen to all these other people in the group, and their situations are so much worse than mine. There's someone in there that's been dealing with this for over twenty years, and they're getting to the end. That's the biggest fear," he says, "the fear of the future."

Bob admits that the meetings aren't always easy for him.

"Judy pressures you a little bit to talk about your feelings. She jumps down my throat, because I won't participate the way she wants me to, so I typed this up for her." He smiles as he hands across a copy of a page he wrote for the meeting. It reads,

> *In an attempt to break down my walls, I am submitting the following:*
>
> *First, I would like to say that my life's experiences have created some very large walls that I have been hiding behind. I feel more comfortable talking to women about my personal life; however, I fear that getting too close to another woman may cause additional complications if that person cannot maintain a strictly "friendship" relationship.*
>
> *I have NEVER cheated on anyone in my life, which my first wife could not say. I love my current wife, and would not do anything to hurt her or her children.*
>
> *One person expressed the following comment which I don't know how to deal with. I was told that they thought I felt "trapped." I guess I do—morally, legally, and financially. I hope this information is helpful in understanding my reluctance to open up with the support group.*

When I look up from reading the paper, Bob is still smiling. He has smiled after almost everything he has said so far. When I ask, "Why are you smiling?" he replies, "I'm not. Sometimes I smile instead of crying."

"I started getting depressed," Bob admits, "and the best way to tell you about that is with a journal I kept. It's all dated." He reaches into his folder and pulls out several more typewritten papers.

Bob may have trouble expressing his feelings in the support group, but the pages he shares show a man who has made a real effort to explore his emotions. Under the heading "Bob's Journal" he has made three columns: one for the date, one for the event, and one marked "Feelings." A review of the journal takes the reader inside Bob's mind . . . .

Date	Event	Feelings
1/12	After spending all day at my mother's funeral, I had been able to hide my feelings until returning home. I told Jean that I needed to be alone for a while and went to have two beers. I was gone approximately two hours. Jean seemed upset and wanted to know what she had done wrong. I stated that she had done nothing wrong and that I just could not be with her 24 hours a day.	I had a very difficult night and felt very sad all morning.
1/13	Jean has a dental appointment tomorrow and a new form is required. I explained that we need to take one copy to the dentist and keep the other copy for a future appointment. This explanation took six tries, and I'm not sure yet if she understands.	I know she cannot help this; however, it troubles me greatly to see her struggle to understand. *I took a depression test on WebMD that showed "moderate" depression.
1/24	In the last few days the person who I was able to talk to and use as a "sounding board" felt we were getting too close and has backed away somewhat. I have found a phone number for a support group and will call them tomorrow.	I have been feeling very sad for the past three days and close to coming to tears.
1/25	Today Jean asked me again how to erase phone calls from her cell phone. I patiently went through the steps several times. Her ability to use the phone is limited to calling and answering only.	I sometimes feel overwhelmed by the repetition of explaining things and the repetitive questions she has.
1/26	In the past two days I have burst into tears for no apparent reason.	Time to contact the doctor!

Bob states that he did see a doctor for his depression. "She put me on pills, but they didn't work. We tried again last month, but the cure was worse than the problem. They didn't work, and the side effects were bad."

He moves his head as if following a bird in flight, then he faces front again and says, "You want me to be totally honest about how I cope with this? I go and have a few beers every day. I can do that now, because I can leave her alone. I know there's going to be a point when I won't be able to leave her alone, and that concerns me a lot. I'm kind of procrastinating, you know? I keep telling myself I'm not to the point yet where I'd have to be with her all the time, or put her in a facility.

"As a matter of fact, one of the nurses at the bar works in a nursing home. I also met somebody there that's a bartender, and her mother's having problems, so her and I—although she works five days a week and can't go to these meetings—I feed her information. We relate to each other because of her problem and my problem."

He describes his wife's mood these days. "She's a very calm person, really, but I know her condition worries her. She's aware she has a problem, and she's becoming very dependent on me. She asks permission to do everything—asking me, 'Is it okay to sit down?' or, 'I'm going to go to the bathroom, is that okay?' It's just continually like that.

"Sometimes I tend to lose my temper a little bit, and after about thirty-some questions I'll say, 'Would you please not ask me any more questions!' and she says things like, 'Well, I'm your biggest problem,' which makes me feel bad.

"We never had any arguments, or fights, or stuff. She's always been insecure, but now she's even more insecure."

I mention to Bob the cards he handed out at the support group meeting with *The Ten Absolutes for Caregivers,* and ask if he refers to the list often.

He smiles and produces one of the cards from his shirt pocket, as if he is never without one.

The card reads:

NEVER ARGUE – Instead – AGREE
NEVER REASON – Instead – DIVERT
NEVER SHAME – Instead – DISTRACT
NEVER LECTURE – Instead – REASSURE
NEVER SAY "REMEMBER" – Instead – REMINISCE
NEVER SAY "I TOLD YOU" – Instead – REPEAT, REGROUP
NEVER SAY "YOU CAN'T" – Instead – SAY "LET'S DO THIS"
NEVER COMMAND/DEMAND – Instead ASK/MODEL
NEVER CONDESCEND – Instead – ENCOURAGE/PRAISE
NEVER FORCE – Instead – REINFORCE

When I ask which item on the list is the most helpful to him, Bob reviews the card and purses his lips. "I can tell you which ones I *don't* do very well with," he says. "It's probably not saying 'I told you.' I violate that quite often. I'll say, 'I told you that an hour ago.'"

He studies the card again, then says, "And the other one is, '*Never reason*.' I always try to reason, and you can't."

When asked which ones he's good at, he's quick to respond.

"'*Never argue*.' I definitely don't argue. I walk away. And I never shame. She'll say, 'It's my fault,' and I'll say, 'It's not your fault.' I never blame her for anything. I don't lecture. I just don't. Sometimes I say, 'Remember?' which you're not supposed to say."

Bob tells me that Jean has a daughter who lives in another state. Communication between the two of them is an issue, but not because of the distance.

"The only way I can talk to her is by email. I can't talk to her on the phone, because she's one of these types," he jabbers with his fingers. "I can't get a word in, so I just communicate by email. I think where she's lacking in understanding is how all of this is affecting me—my mental state, which is . . . ." He waggles his hand in place of saying "*iffy*."

"I'm depressed. I'm frustrated. And that's another thing that came up in a group meeting. They jumped on me. They said, 'You're not angry?' I said, 'No, I'm not angry. I'm frustrated.' Judy and two others said, 'You've gotta be angry.' I said, 'No I'm not angry; I'm frustrated with the continual questions and the repeating of everything.'"

More recent entries in his journal make this clear:

Date	Event	Feelings
4/25	*I am seeing a decrease in Jean's ability to comprehend. She seems to be confused with basic things like spring, summer, winter, and fall, and she asks repeatedly when each starts.*	*I am going to the support group meetings weekly. They help me cope much better than if I did not go.*
4/27	*Yesterday on the way to my veterans' meeting, Jean was trying to remember some of the members' names. After about 30 questions, I said, "Please, no more questions."*	*I know she is struggling, but I feel like I'm being dragged into her world of confusion.*

Bob continues talking about his stepdaughter.

"Her idea of helping is sending some money every once in a while. I'm looking for moral support . . . encouragement . . . that type of thing, and that isn't there."

When asked how his stepdaughter could provide more support, he smiles. "By spending time with her mother. More time— not just three or four times a year."

He is quick to add, "I would like to say that she means well, but she just doesn't know how to give the kind of help I need. If she were here more often, I would feel like I wasn't left alone so much. We would be sharing responsibility, not . . . ." His voice drifts off, then he says, "She keeps saying, 'We're a team,' but it's only a team with what she wants to do. She calls quite often. She does call her mother every few days, but she's a team member from a distance."

When asked how he copes on his own, Bob replies, "One day at a time. One hour at a time. One minute at a time." He shrugs, and smiles. "Standard answer."

He points to the latest entries in his journal, indicating that I should read them:

Date	Event	Feelings
5/22	*I have now been off Zoloft (anti-depressant) for 30 days.*	*The feelings of anxiety have returned, and I am on the verge of tears often. Tonight was especially bad, and I called a friend just to give me a hug over the phone.*
5/29	*Today, for some reason, I was extremely agitated, and Jean kept asking me the usual "twenty questions." I was so agitated and nervous, I just said "I'm going to take a motorcycle ride and I will be back later."*	*I rode my bike for about 70 miles and felt better when I returned around noon.*
5/30	*Today, Memorial Day, we had our support group meeting. As our facilitator stated, "Alzheimer's does not take a Holiday." In the meeting I reluctantly relayed the information above about how I was doing. The members of the support group congratulated me for beginning to open up with my true feelings and we had lunch together.*	*The group is very concerned about my mental state.*
5/31	*When I told my stepdaughter how I was feeling, she immediately told me that I was threatening her by indicating that I may have to go in the hospital for mental health reasons, which would require her to take care of her mother for up to six weeks.*	*I blew up and stated to her that I was not threatening her, only stating the facts. I told her that I was on the brink of a mental break-down and I will not have a comment again until I cool off. I then hung up.*

6/1	*My stepdaughter called back four times on my cell phone, which I ignored. I later retrieved the messages she left me, and she apologized for upsetting me. She said I should have told her how I felt and the seriousness of the situation.*	*If I have trouble opening up to the receptive, understanding support group with my personal feelings, how am I supposed to open up to a person with this kind of attitude?*

I finish reading Bob's journal and look across the table at him. His eyes speak of the pain and frustration that he expresses quite clearly with his written words, but those feelings have yet to reach the rest of his face.

In spite of his feelings—or perhaps, as he has stated, to avoid them—Bob Jameson is still smiling.

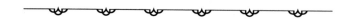

"Barb, you're next," says Judy. "What's going on in your life?"

Barb clears her throat, then begins. "For those of you who don't know, Jack is in a home now." She turns away and stares at the wall for a moment. When she looks back, her eyes are moist.

"We were discussing how many times I come to visit him during the week. I'm still coming to grips with the fact that I do that for me; I don't do that for him. He probably doesn't understand whether I'm there or not there. He told someone the other day after I'd been there every day for five days that I don't come to see him anymore, so it's like aaaaaggggghhh!" She turns her fingers into claws and makes a monster face.

"Another time when I was gone for a week, he said, 'Well, when you were here yesterday....'"

"*That's very common,*" Judy says. "*You don't need to go every day. It's good for you to have time for yourself.*"

Barb's mouth twists. "*Rationally, I know that, but the distance between the head and the heart is so far. I'm still trying to shorten that distance. So that's where I'm at.*"

"*You're doing great,*" Judy says. "*Just hang in there.*"

17

Still a Person

Outsiders will tell you that Arbor Village Rehabilitation and Nursing Center is not the Taj Mahal. The cinder block construction is visible on some of the interior walls. The architecture is dated. These and other material aspects of the facility lose their importance, however, after only a few minutes in the French Quarter—the name selected for the Alzheimer's Unit by those who live and work there. The happy feeling engendered by the colorful New Orleans mural just inside the locked double doors is reflected in the smiling faces of the staff.

The attitude of Belinda Brine, LPN, the unit manager of "Bourbon Street"—one of two Alzheimer's wings at Arbor Village—explains why she and her fellow staff members smile so much.

"I love my work. I've been there for seventeen years, and I wouldn't be there this long if I didn't," Belinda says. "I just love taking care of the people who can't care for themselves. That's why I went into nursing. I love elderly people. Some of them have so many interesting stories to share. I'm also fascinated by how the mind works and the things that can happen to the mind with different diseases."

She admits that she calls the patients "my babies."

"I'm very protective of my residents. They're like our family. A lot of our employees spend more time there than we do at home. Many of the residents don't have families that visit, so we become their family, and we don't want anything to happen to them. We make sure their needs are met."

She explains that "we" includes her staff of three to four Certified Nursing Assistants. They have their hands full taking care of their twenty-eight "babies."

"My shift is from six-forty-five until three-fifteen," she says, "and every day is different. It's like working in a circus. You never know what's going to happen from day to day. Behaviors vary. It could be calm and quiet one day, and totally off the wall the next. You could have people fighting with each other—both verbally and physically—or residents refusing care, and all of that can have a domino effect.

"It's a lot of mental work," Belinda says, then she admits, "Sometimes I take it home with me, but I have a wonderful husband. He listens, and he doesn't judge. He leaves me alone when I need to be alone. There are times when I go home and say, 'Okay everybody, just give me a half an hour,' then I just recoup and regenerate."

The demands at work and the desire to not take work home with her explain why Nurse Brine requested to meet at a local Denny's Restaurant to talk. We sit on the patio and chat without distractions. She appears tense, and explains that it is only because of the interview. If there is pressure at work, it doesn't show on her face. With her long, brown hair and stylish glasses, she looks a good ten years younger than her age, hardly old enough to be the grandmother that she is.

"I work seven days a week," she says, "five days a week at my job, and two days a week caring for the other end of the spectrum." She is referring to her grandchildren: an eight-month-old, a four-year-old and an eight-year-old.

"I helped deliver the youngest one," she says proudly.

After showing me the children's photos and exchanging a few more pleasantries, I ask her to describe a typical day on her unit. She takes a sip from a glass of iced tea, then answers, "In the morning the residents get up, and we assist those who need help. There are some we actually have to lift out of bed, and there are others for whom we just have to open the door and tell them it's time for breakfast. They'll get up and take care of toileting and dressing themselves."

She is quick to clarify, "We have a few that can dress themselves, and a few who think they can. They'll come out with two dresses and pants, but we let them wear what they want. It's their home. The only thing we frown on is if they come out naked.

"So we brush their teeth, clean them up, and get them dressed. All of the staff will help feed them breakfast—anybody that's able to pass trays and feed will chip in. We have four different dining rooms on our unit, with one that's called 'fine dining.' The residents who don't need as much assistance eat in there. They're a little more aware of their surroundings. The ones that require more assistance eat in the three dining rooms on the unit.

"After breakfast they're toileted again. Some of them know enough to ask for the bathroom, but they have to be shown where the bathroom is because they forget from day to day. There's one in each room, and in the TV area, and another in each dining area except for the fine dining."

Belinda explains that the CNAs do most of the hands-on care. "I give them their medication. That's my job: medications and treatments. The CNAs will let me know if they need help. They usually buddy up, though, because a lot of the residents take two people to do things.

"After breakfast some go to therapy and some stay on the unit. We just interact with them all day—reading them the newspaper, talking, dancing . . . . They love to dance—even the ones in wheelchairs. They just move their hands and swing back and forth." She rocks her body from side to side.

"Some of them like to watch TV," she continues. "Some wander down to the other unit and visit. Some go outside. We have a nice area where residents can go outside. It's not usual for a nursing home to have a place like that, especially in a secured environment, but we have two different courtyards they can go out to. There's a walkway that goes all the way around each courtyard, so even if they're in a wheelchair they can go outside.

"There are little garden areas where they can do gardening." She smiles. "They pull up the plants and plant them again, and some of them bring the plants inside. They'll go outside when it's raining, and we'll get an umbrella and go and retrieve them." She says this as if it's no imposition.

"After their morning activity, the ones that need help are toileted again. They have lunch, then some of them lie down and take a nap. We have to assist those who can't get into bed themselves, but if they're tired and want to lie down, we let them. We get to know pretty much the ones that want that. That's where we're like their family. We get to know what they need without asking.

"Most of them will sleep right until suppertime, and we have different activities going on all day. Sundays they have church services in the main dining room. Most of the activities are in there, and they'll mingle with other residents who don't have dementia.

"After they have dinner, you still have residents that are going to therapy or activities. Then they get showers and get ready for bed. They're on a schedule for showers three days a week, and we break it up between the seven-to-three and three-to-eleven shift. They get a bed bath every day," she stresses, "but they actually go into the shower three days a week."

If her day seems routine, Belinda quickly dispels that idea.

"It's not usually boring on our unit," she says, laughing. "You never know what's going to happen. We might have a resident that we have a hard time getting under control. That gets the other residents upset. Then you might have incidents of people falling, or a resident might strike out, and then you have people fighting.

"There are days that I don't get a break. That's when you have to use humor just to get through the shift. That's one thing the staff does say to each other, 'You gotta laugh,' especially when we have people acting up and getting everybody else upset. Some get upset easily.

"We can always tell when the regular staff has been off, because some of the residents act up more for people they don't know. They might refuse to take their medications or refuse ADL care." She explains that ADL stands for Activities of Daily Living, a nice way of saying that they might be wet and need changing.

"They have a right to refuse their care or their medication, so we try to encourage them to accept our help. Some of the answers we get are funny, like, 'I don't want the medicine. You take it!' Then it gets to a point where we just have to give them their care, whether or not they cooperate. There's a fine line between neglect and abuse," she says, "and you have to learn where that line is.

"We have some residents that can have attitudes. Sometimes you just have to leave them alone, but we can't do that all the time. Certain things might trigger their moods, and we have medication that helps with that. Some of them need to be medicated more often than others, but that's usually a last resort. We try to redirect them. We try to get them involved in something else to change their thought process. Sometimes it works, and sometimes it doesn't.

"You have to kind of get in their world," she says, "and try to find out what they're thinking. We try to approach them in a calm way. Sometimes just a touch will calm them. We have some dolls that were donated, and the residents like to hold and cuddle the babies. We do have one gentleman who thinks the baby is his." She laughs. "That creates a problem, because he doesn't want to eat until the baby has eaten."

"I have one gentleman who follows me around all day long," she says. "He thinks I'm his wife sometimes. So I let him follow me if that gives him comfort."

Belinda states that the staff will go above and beyond the norm to make their patients feel at home. "There was one patient who was constantly trying to get out of the facility," she says. "He kept trying to climb the fence, because he had to get home to take care of his animals."

The solution was unique: "We brought the animals to him." This explains the two goats that permanently reside in a yard next to the residents' fenced-in courtyard.

"Debbie got him the goats," Belinda says, referring to Arbor Village's administrator, Debbie Brazill. "They've been there a couple of years. The resident's son actually brought them in. His father walked outside, and the first thing he said was, 'Those aren't my animals,' but he would go out and spend a little time with them. After a while he kind of ignored them, but we kept them anyway."

I ask who takes care of the goats.

Belinda laughs. "I believe the Activities Department does, because when we found out we were getting goats, I said, 'Goats are not in my job description.'"

I ask what her biggest challenge is as the unit manager.

"Dealing with the families," she answers without hesitation. "Some of them haven't accepted the disease. For instance, I've had one resident for a couple of years, and sometimes he doesn't realize who his wife is. He might be holding the hand of another woman, and that upsets his wife. So, they're not accepting of the fact that their loved one is not intentionally doing that.

"I know it's hard. They didn't ask for their loved one to be afflicted with Alzheimer's. You're married to someone for years, then all of a sudden you see them holding hands or kissing someone else. I try to explain to them a bit about the disease process and how it affects the mind. I encourage them to join a support group. It's good for them to talk to other people who've been in that situation, and find out how they handle it.

"I tell them they can't stop living their life. Most of the caregivers have taken care of their loved one longer than they really should. It starts to affect their health and their mental well-being."

We discuss the nursing home stigma, and whether that may cause some people to delay putting their loved one in a home. Some feel uncomfortable being around so many patients with dementia, or they may be put off by the unpleasant smells in a nursing home.

Belinda shrugs this off. "We're just used to it," she says. "It's no different than taking care of a baby. They're people. They're human beings that have a disease.

"People who are uncomfortable with the nursing home environment should come and visit," she advises. "Come volunteer. We have some family members who bring their children in, and they'll volunteer with the activities throughout the day. I think a lot of the younger people need to be more aware of what it's really like.

"We have such a caring staff. Some of the CNAs that work with me have been there as long as I have. You have to enjoy that kind of work, or you need to get another job, because it's very stressful.

But I think a lot of the families—if they spend any time there—can actually see how the staff cares for the residents.

"It's not like in the hospital where you have a revolving door with them coming and going," Belinda says. "The ones we have are there to stay with us. I've had people as long as seven or eight years, and as short as a month. Most of mine are long-term. We get pretty close to some of them, and that's okay. You have to earn their trust and build a relationship with them.

"It's funny," she says, smiling, "because some of the most difficult patients we've had in the past are the ones we miss the most when they're gone. I honestly don't know why that is. I guess it livens up the unit a little bit.

"So many of them still have a lot to share. They still have needs that have to be met. They still know how to be affectionate," she says, "and they still want to be loved."

And with great simplicity, Nurse Belinda Brine summarizes what she has learned from seventeen years of working with her babies:

"They're still a person," she says, as if it's the most obvious thing in the world, and then she repeats, "they're still a person."

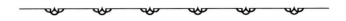

Judy gives a "your turn" nod to a woman in a red sweater. The woman takes a deep breath, and as she exhales, her face turns the same shade as her sweater. She shakes her head as if to clear it, then says, "I'm Carol Sue, and my husband's in a nursing home now, too. I beat myself up at Christmas, and I couldn't stop this." She sweeps her hands in front of her face to indicate her crying.

"I took him out to dinner on Christmas Day, but I got sick with a sinus infection. I usually go to visit him every day, but I couldn't go for five days because I was sick. I called all the time."

Carol Sue wipes roughly at her tears. "Anyhow, when I went in on Wednesday, he said, 'I thought I'd never see you again!' I felt so guilty."

Her voice chokes on the last word, and she stops for a moment to get herself together. When she regains her voice, she says, "I had my meal there with him, and we were sitting there afterwards. They had some activity going on, and he said, 'You know, we have a pretty good life.'"

"I thought, 'You know, he went full circle.' He forgot all about me not coming to visit, so this is good. I'm not crying anymore. I came today because I wasn't going to cry."

She laughs at herself and the group laughs with her—big laughs that are filled with understanding.

"That's okay," Judy says, smiling. "This is the place that you come to cry. It's all right."

"So that was my holiday," Carol Sue says, turning her palms outward. "I'm glad it's over."

18

BREATHTAKING RESULTS

IT IS NINE A.M. AND DEBBIE BRAZILL is the personification of "perky." Her long, brown hair is still damp from a swim at the local Y as she welcomes me to Arbor Village Rehabilitation and Nursing Center with a broad smile and sparkling eyes. Her hands are thin and feminine like the rest of her, but there is great strength in her handshake. Her voice is high-pitched—almost childlike for a woman in her forties—but she exudes confidence and warmth.

She has just arrived at work, and already a voice squawks through the speaker of a multi-line telephone on her desk. She winces and pushes a button on the phone, switching it to silent mode. She starts to sit, then with a shake of her curly locks, comes out from behind her large desk and takes the chair beside me. We chat for a few minutes to get to know each other, then get down to business.

I ask her to describe her job, and she replies, "I'm the administrator here, and what that really means is . . . ."

Her voice drifts off for a moment as she reconsiders her response.

"Everybody thinks I run the place," she says, "but I really don't. I coordinate. I enable the staff. I'm kind of the wind beneath their wings so they can stay in flight."

I ask how she became an administrator.

"I have the same degree as everybody else," she says, "hospital administration. But I grew up in nursing homes. When I was thirteen years old I started as a part-time receptionist at a nursing home near my house. I would ride my bicycle to work with all of my activities in my backpack for the residents to do. I had the biggest activity center in the building up at the front desk in the lobby."

I ask how she was able to get a job at such a young age. She lowers her eyes, and admits, "I lied about my age." The ensuing giggle shows that she harbors no guilt about the deception.

"My family needed the money," she shrugs, "so I had to go to work. At the time it was just a job, but then I stayed because I fell in love with them. I fell in love with the geriatrics—with the residents.

"They have such a wealth of information," she says, "but I hated the fact that this one wanted a bath, but it wasn't their bath day, so they couldn't get a bath. I mean, how would you feel if you're used to taking a bath every day, and you didn't get a bath because it's not your day? Now you only get one twice a week, so what do you do? And they get you up when you're not used to getting up, or it's nine o'clock at night and you're supposed to go to bed. They would come to my desk in the lobby because they didn't want to go to bed then."

She shakes her head at the memories.

"You get up at a different time than I get up. You want something different for breakfast than I do. You might like showers, and I like baths . . . . I don't want the residents to be institutionalized when they get here. I want it to be that when you come here, nothing changes but your address. All of these things are part of the culture change movement."

She explains, "Culture change is being led by a group of forward-thinking individuals and pioneers in the nursing home field who are out to change the world in nursing home care. It's been around since '96 or '97. There's an overall national Pioneer Network, and there's a chapter for each state."

Debbie reveals that she serves on the Florida board of the Pioneer Network. She recommends that anyone looking for a nursing home for a loved one visit the Pioneer Network website for a list of questions to ask when considering a potential home.[5]

As part of culture change at Arbor Village, Debbie describes how the facility is divided both geographically and functionally into

5   See www.PioneerNetwork.org

what the staff calls "neighborhoods," with twenty to thirty residents in each.

"The neighborhood known as 'the French Quarter' is the secure unit for our residents with Alzheimer's. On one side are the folks that are walking around, and on the other side are the folks that are in wheelchairs, although they mix and mingle a little bit. But they're all confused folks over there," she says with a gentle smile. "Then we have another unit that's very short-term rehab, then a longer-term rehab, which is for people recovering from stroke or those with generalized weakness."

"All of the neighborhoods operate somewhat independently," she explains, "so they have a neighborhood council and neighborhood meetings, and they have an elected mayor, who could be anybody. Some of the neighborhoods have residents that are neighbors, and some of the neighborhoods have a housekeeper who's a neighbor, or it could be an activity leader. It depends on the neighborhood."

A pair of birds chirps loudly from the hallway as I ask how long she has been the administrator.

"I've been here seven years," she says. "I'm part owner. The other owner is my partner. The previous owners went bankrupt, and the place was sold at auction.

"It used to be named We Care, but the local EMS folks called it We Scare because it was so bad. The building was falling down. The residents didn't get bathed, and it smelled really bad." She makes a face. "Call lights were going off from the residents needing help in their rooms, and the CNAs would just sit around. It was your standard nursing home horror story.

"So we went to the auction, and it had such a bad reputation that I told the man I went with, 'I'll never be the administrator at We Care!'"

She rolls her eyes, then looks around at her office.

"Words I'll eat," she says, with laughter that sounds like mini hiccups.

"So we go to auction and we're completely unprepared. We didn't have any paperwork drawn up. We put in a bid for the auction and we got the building. And then I said, 'Uh oh!' And he said, 'Now you're going to be the administrator!'

"So we changed the name. We really needed to change the name. Arbor Village was the name of a wing over here—their rehab wing. People already were somewhat familiar with it and it didn't have a bad reputation associated with it."

She reaches down and smoothes the hem of her bright print dress.

"I came over with a team. I worked at a place half the size—a hundred and twenty beds—just ten miles down the road. When I left there, nine department heads came with me and forty-two employees."

I ask how her previous employer felt about her depleting their staff so drastically.

"They hated me!" she says, but her laughter reveals no regrets as she adds, "They had my poster on the wall like Osama bin Laden!

"We had all been together for years, and we're still together. We had work to do, and I needed their help. I didn't do a whole lot of recruiting. They all said, 'We've got a good team. We know what to expect, and we know your management style.' So we all came together.

"The people who already worked here said it was like a tidal wave hit." She grins, then adds, "And they're still feeling the waves seven years later!"

We discuss how much nurse Belinda Brine and the CNAs who work in the Alzheimer's unit love their work. They do not sound like the CNAs that Debbie saw working at We Care in the old days, and I ask what brought about the change in attitude.

She puts her hands out as if the answer is obvious. "You empower them. You give them the ability to make decisions on their own. You don't tell them what to do. They *know* what to do. They are front line staff and they are tired of idiots above them telling them, 'Oh no, you've gotta do it this way,' or 'Oh no, you've gotta do it that way.'

"All of the residents are individuals," she says. "You have to take care of them differently, depending on their needs. The top-down make-a-rule doesn't work for everyone. It might work for Mary Jane, but it doesn't work for Bob. So, you ask the CNAs to write care plans based on what they tell us is the best way to take care of Bob so that other CNAs that are floating or new will have their expertise."

Debbie explains that the culture change hasn't come without some resistance. "It's hard to get department heads to let go of control. Nurses are very, 'follow doctor's orders, gotta do exactly what it says.' So that's why I've drilled into them, 'You know, it's great that they get their medicine, but it's even better if you can sit down and talk to them.'

"You instill that philosophy every day," she says. "You do it through your policy and procedures, and by changing the way you do things."

By way of example, she tells how they used a grant from the government for an innovative initiative.

"We put kitchenettes in all the neighborhoods. Now we have five little kitchens, and each one has permanently assigned cooks. That's the only kitchen they work in, and the CNAs in that neighborhood are the only CNAs the cooks converse with. The residents are the only residents they cook for.

"Usually you have one big kitchen, and the cooks never see the residents or the CNAs. The cooks never come out of that kitchen. You have one cook who will cook for two hundred and ten residents, and they see nothing but a meal ticket. They don't know that Mrs. Jones, 'Oh, I think she's getting tired of scrambled eggs today,' which is what these cooks know. These cooks know that Mrs. Jones likes her oatmeal with peanut butter and honey. They know it because they know the residents."

She realizes that she has been gesturing quite dramatically and presses one hand onto the other as if to tame it. "I'm Italian. I talk with my hands," she says, laughing sheepishly, but her face is full of pride as she continues bragging about her staff.

"They have to get out and take their orders and find out what they want. That idea came from the staff—from all over the neighborhoods. They learn from each other. They talk to each other. Right now we're looking at turning all the little dining areas into five-star dining. The neighborhoods are competing against each other in nice friendly competition, so they're all going out and getting decorations, and getting nice tablecloths.

"They want to get the best music and the best little sound system so all of the residents have the fine dining experience. Some of them have asked me to print real restaurant menus. It's all about empowering the employees to make those decisions."

Debbie proves that culture change works by sharing the example of a management trainee who recently began working at Arbor Village. "She went out and interviewed the residents about potential improvements. She came back and said, 'People are really happy here. I mean, they are *really* happy. I can't get them to tell me anything that's wrong!'

"We still have to meet regulations. We still have to be clean. We still have to meet infection control. Our standards of care have to be high, but that doesn't mean we can't have a good quality of life, too."

When asked to describe quality of life initiatives in the Alzheimer's unit, Debbie Brazill responds without hesitation.

"The difference is permanently and consistently assigned staff members that know the residents and love them. Let me tell you, you cannot move these CNAs. They're not going anywhere. They're not working anywhere else. They're not going to another unit."

She gazes in the direction of the French Quarter, then says, "Sometimes they need to go out and take a breather for ten minutes if they have a rough group, but they get right back in there. They worry about them when they're on vacation. They'll call and find out what's going on.

"You can tell the quality of life is good just seeing the residents' smiles, seeing them interact and seeing them not zombified. A lot of times the residents on an Alzheimer's unit will have a very high psychotropic antipsychotic drug use. In fact," she says, sitting up taller, "I just went over our drug use, and our facility is lower than the average for the entire state of Florida because we keep our residents busy. That's called keeping them 'meaningfully engaged.' We try and find things that they like to do and that they want to do, even if it's for just five minutes at a time. Sometimes that's the extent of their attention span, but it's that five minutes that helps."

Debbie continues talking about the culture change. "I have management staff out there in the glassed-in TV room in the Alzheimer's unit. There are desks for our social worker and our Minimum Data Set Assessor right inside there so they can see what's going on and be available. They're there to talk to the residents and help out when needed.

"I see them at lunchtime out there helping to pass trays. If somebody's been outside too long, they go out and help get them back in. When they see that a resident is especially agitated, running up and down the hall, and the CNAs or the nurse is unavailable, they can come out and say, 'Hey . . . .' It's very helpful.

"In a normal nursing home, those staff members would be in an office with a door. It was our idea to put them out there in the middle, and they love it."

She stops for a moment and reconsiders her words. "At first, though," she tilts her head, "at first I got a lot of, 'I can't work out here! The residents take all my paper, they take my stapler, the telephone's gone when I get back!' And then there was the resident who rolled up all the papers from one of the desks and fed them to the goats." She puts a hand to her mouth and giggles. "I would admit that it's probably a tough work environment," she says, with no sign of sympathy.

"It's good for the residents to have them so available," she says with a shrug, "and the two who work out there love it now. They're probably not as productive as they would be in an office, but they're available for the families and the residents."

She sits back and crosses her legs. "I love this place. There's a funny story every day. We used to have a resident on the Alzheimer's unit who danced with Queen Elizabeth. That was his job. He was her paid escort."

I ask her to clarify if the man had merely imagined this unusual job, and Debbie shakes her head.

"We have all kinds of pictures of him with the queen, complete with signatures and little notes from her. He was a wonderful dancer. They never forget how to dance. We play music every day back there for the residents to dance, and they come in and they'll dance with you." She tilts her head and quips, "But I'm not as good a dancer as the queen."

She then relates the story of a resident who used to be the director of nursing at a neighboring facility.

"She was wandering around and she went outside in the fenced-in area. She couldn't find the door back in, even though all the sidewalks lead to the door. She started taking a screen out of the window of one of the other residents on the unit so she could get back in. We have another resident who used to be a police officer, and he goes out and points his finger at her. 'I've been watching you!' Debbie says in a deep voice, mimicking the former police officer. 'I knew this was going to happen!' he said, and he arrested her!"

She laughs in a series of short giggles that leave her curls bouncing.

"That same resident was also an auctioneer later in life, and he just sold the piano in the dining room for twenty-one thousand dollars." She chuckles. "He auctioned it off. People were in there eating, and he just stood up, all impromptu, and in that auctioneer's voice he sold it. The residents were all bidding! I was there and I said, 'If we can get twenty-one thousand for that piano, they can have it!'"

We shift gears and talk for a few minutes about the negative image many outsiders have of nursing homes.

Debbie shakes her head. "See, I'm not coming from that. I've been in nursing homes so long that I don't remember what it's like to come in and be uncomfortable when you see these unusual things and smell the unusual smells.

"Placing a loved one in a nursing home is probably one of the best decisions a caretaker can make," Debbie says. "They think they're doing the right thing by keeping them home, and I applaud that, but if they put them in a place that's as much like home as it can possibly be, when the caregivers are here they are rested. They're not impatient and they can spend real quality time just paying attention to their loved one.

"When you're with them twenty-four hours a day, you don't appreciate them as much. Here they have so many other people that have so much to offer them, and everybody's giving them their best. They don't get an impatient word. They don't get a 'No, don't do that! Stop that!' Here they can wander anywhere they want to.

"We have so many Alzheimer's patients that come in because they broke a hip. They get so aggravated on the rehabilitation unit because they go out a door and somebody's dragging them back in. Somebody's always telling them no. Once they get mobile, we immediately put them on the Alzheimer's unit. In there they can do whatever they want. The doors to the unit are all secure, but there are doors that lead outside to fenced-in areas. They can go out one door, and they come right back in the other."

She wrinkles her nose and begins to share another story. "It was so cute the other day. I was out walking around—"

I interrupt to ask why she was walking around.

"Why?" she asks. "I wander around." She shrugs. "I'm lost like they are."

I'm curious if she was deliberately practicing a proven leadership technique known as Management by Walking Around—a technique used by managers who care enough to get out of their offices and take the pulse of their workplace.

"Yeah," she says with a modest wave of her hand, then quickly changes the subject back to her story.

"So I went into this woman's room and there she is by the bed. She's got one of the cloth napkins from the dining room, and she's packin' up." Debbie lowers her voice conspiratorially. "She's puttin' stuff in it," she says, mimicking the woman placing things one by one on the napkin. "She's putting her lotion, and her nail clippers, and her brush, and her toothbrush, and she's got it all in this little sack like a hitchhiker. She has her going-out hat on, and she looks up at me and she goes, 'Shhhhh!'" Debbie places a finger to her lips.

"She heads out the door, and I follow her. Her door is one of the last ones at the end of the hallway, which goes out, but it's to a secure yard. So she goes toward the door with her little pack, and she looks both ways, and *voom*! —she goes out the door like she's getting away. She's going somewhere! She's getting away! She's sneaking out! But we know she's secure, so we don't have to go chase her.

"A few minutes later I see her coming in the other door, and she's just fine. She got it all out of her system. She ran away, and she came back, and nobody had to say anything to her. Nobody had to chase her down. Nobody said, 'No, you can't do that!'

"How many residents have we had admitted because they were lost for hours?" she asks, frowning. "And that's got to be scary. But here they can sneak out and they come right back in the other door, because all the sidewalks go in circles!

"We take the Alzheimer's residents out to lunch three times a month. We take twenty-two at a time. We have multiple staff members and volunteers with them. The Alzheimer's Association pays for two of those times, and we take them out another time and pay for it.

"At first I was a little leery about taking all these Alzheimer's patients out, so I would drive my personal van and I would take the six who would come with me. The first time they couldn't figure out how to get in the back seat. They'd sit on the arm, so I'd have to guide them in. About the fourth time I had to take a phone call, and they all got in on their own and sat in their seats just fine. So there is some learning that can occur."

It is obvious that she and her staff get close to the residents. Knowing that most of the Alzheimer's residents spend their final days at the home, I ask how the staff deals with their deaths.

"We have a little vigil that we put on for each one that passes away. We light a candle for them. We put their name in the chapel, and we celebrate their life. The staff and the other residents talk about them. At the neighborhood meeting we have a moment of silence. It is tough, but you realize that things change."

I mention that many caregivers find visiting their loved ones in a home very painful, especially when the loved one cries at the end of a visit.

Debbie nods with understanding. "Yes, and two minutes after the family member walks out the door, they don't remember they were there. It's very hard, but they don't cry anymore.

"They do this number," she says and waves goodbye. "They watch them leave, then we tell them, 'Hey, let's go listen to the music, Martha.' They say, 'Okay!' and off they go. That's it.

"But it's absolutely worthwhile to visit them," she emphasizes, "even if they don't remember them visiting. It's good for the caregiver and it's good for the resident. Talk to them about memories. Make them feel alive. That's important. There are some people that don't have Alzheimer's who don't feel alive. Let them continue to be alive, to feel things.

"They still have emotions and they still have needs. They still need somebody to hug them, to hold their hand, to laugh with them, to cry with them. They still have all their emotions. They might not understand their emotions, but they're still a real person."

She points a finger. "Now, they might not be the person that their loved one remembers, but the family member still brings back memories for them. They still have memories.

"Sometimes families will come in and say, 'Mom, what did you have for breakfast?'"

She sighs. "For an Alzheimer's patient, that's one of the worst things you can ask them. They don't remember, and they don't want to tell you they don't remember, because that makes them feel inadequate. And so you can say things like, 'Mom, you remember when I was a little girl and we tie-dyed those shirts, and we got dye all over the place?'

"They remember stuff like that." In a sing-songy voice she gives another example. "'Remember that story you used to tell about you and your sister picking blackberries and all the prickers all over?'

"Bring back things that they'll remember so they feel like they're able to do something. If we keep reminding them of their disabilities, then they'll forget about their abilities, and they still have a lot of abilities."

She takes a deep breath. "I know they're raising all this money to try and find a cure for Alzheimer's, but I think they need to put a lot more money into helping people cope with the disease. They put out checklists to put them in stages, but then what do you do? So, she's in stage five. Good. Now what? It's not helpful.

"You find out what they're able to still do, and you allow them to do it. On the Alzheimer's unit we cook, and people say, 'Oh my gosh, you give them knives?'

She juts out her chin and says, "I sure do. Sometimes after they cook it, it's not edible, but that's okay, too!" She laughs, then grows serious. "The point is to go to their abilities. They're still able to chop up those carrots. They're still able to peel the cucumbers. They're still able to make a salad. They make egg salad over there. They make deviled eggs. They make pigs in a blanket. It makes them feel like they've done something. It boosts their self-esteem. They are still capable of doing things.

"If somebody puts you in a chair and takes care of you every day for the rest of your life, how do you feel?" She throws her hands out, then she gives a forlorn look at the pile of papers on her desk. "I mean, it might be good for a few days, let me tell you, but after a few weeks, now what do you do? I mean, 'I'm going to sit here, and you're just waiting for me to die.' That's how they feel.

"So you have to give them some responsibilities. We have some residents who set the table and they clear the table. They might be clearing the table before people finish eating, but it's okay!" She grins and giggles some more.

As the interview comes to an end, I pick up an Arbor Village brochure and point to a phrase that stands out from the others: *"When we work at our highest levels, the results are **breathtaking.**"* The word is highlighted and jumps off the page. It is not an adjective that one would normally associate with a nursing home.

Debbie rocks her head back and forth, seemingly embarrassed, but obviously pleased.

"A team of my employees put that together. I love the brochure, but I didn't know if people would understand it. To us it means that it's amazing what you can do when you all work together and you work at your moral and ethical high. It's breathtaking when you do what you feel is the right thing to do, not what all these regulations tell you that you have to do.

"I have such a problem, because I go out with the Pioneer Network, and I do speaking engagements for them. Talking to some of the corporations . . . ." She shakes her head at the bureaucrats she has to deal with. "Yeah. How do you run a chain of facilities with culture change?

"You can tell the attitude of the staff in some of the places where they need help," she says. "They've grown hardened. But here, the staff is happy. They have a say in how they do their jobs and what's the best way. They want to do a good job. People are basically good. They want to do well. This is not a place that people go to work to get an easy buck." She blows a puff of air through her lips and adds, "You can make a whole lot more money somewhere else doing a whole lot less labor.

"The corporate places think the way I manage is with no rules because I don't make each neighborhood follow the same procedure for everything. I say, 'No, it empowers the staff. For kitchen preparation, for example, the way they get their meals out is different for each neighborhood. The folks on the orthopedic and cardiac units are short-term. They tell you what they want, and they want it now. With the people in the Alzheimer's unit, you have to put food in front of them as they sit down to eat, or they're going forget that they're there to eat. If the food's not there right away, they're going to think they already ate, and get up and leave!"

She laughs at this image of the residents that she has come to love, and says, "We still have a ways to go. It's always a work in progress. Always. It's a journey."

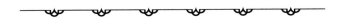

The next person to speak stands out for two reasons: he is one of the few men at the support group meeting, and at fifty-something, he is younger than most others in the room.

"My name's Dave," he announces. "My mother has been in Arbor Village for about five months. Her anger has increased substantially. She gets pretty mean, and that's tough.

"Last Sunday I spent two and half hours with her, and I was only home twenty minutes before she called and said, 'Where the hell are you? You haven't been here!'" He shakes his head. "It's amazing that she can dial a phone with the numbers rubbed off."

He fidgets in his seat, then says, "She's got some crazy stories. The floor in the home is nice and shiny, and she thinks she's drowning. If they have rain, she thinks she's going to drown."

"Some of them are very afraid of water," Judy informs the group. "You can't even get them near a bathtub or a shower."

"Yeah, it's amazing," Dave says. "Other than that, when I leave to go home, it's pretty tough."

Judy asks, "What do you say to her when you leave?"

He shrugs. "I just say, 'See you tomorrow.' I'm here six days a week for an hour and a half minimum."

"So, you don't use the word 'home'?"

"No. I say, 'I'm going to leave and eat' or 'I have to go home and eat." He catches himself and smiles. "Yeah, I use the word 'home.'"

"Don't ever use the word' home," Judy advises. "Tell her you have to go to the Laundromat. Tell her you have

to go to the bank. Whatever. When you use the word 'home,' you put that back in their head, and it makes it a lot worse."

"It's gotten to the point now where she really cries. I mean really bad, like a baby. So I say, 'Gotta go, gotta go,' and you just have to leave. One of the nurses will say, 'You'd better just go. She doesn't even know you're here,' but the constant crying, the name-calling, the constant nastiness has gotten a lot worse."

"What was her personality like when she was, quote, 'normal,'" Judy asks, adding, "Whatever 'normal' is?"

Dave shakes his head. "All the kids in the neighborhood loved her. I don't think I ever heard her say a cuss word. Ever." He chokes up, and appears embarrassed by his emotion. "It's tough."

Judy gives him a gentle smile. "That's okay, Dave. It must be terrible to have to be your father to your mother."

He presses his thumb and index finger to his eyes, then says, "I'm sorry."

"No. Don't be sorry," Judy says as someone passes him a box of Kleenex. "What I was trying to get at is, we all understand that you're dealing with a beautiful person that's become ill, you know? But you're a good son. Hang in there."

"I'm working on it," he says.

"Do you take her down to the ice cream shop they have at Arbor Village?"

He gives a single shake of his head. "A lot of times she doesn't want to leave her room."

"Does she have a baby doll or a stuffed animal?"

"Nah. I think when you bring her stuff, she really doesn't remember."

"But you know what?" Judy says, leaning forward in her chair. "Women never forget that they were mothers. Somewhere inside them that's still there, and they will

hang onto those babies when they don't have anything else."

The woman to Dave's left says, "I noticed that some new babies showed up on the Alzheimer's unit this morning. It was so sweet, because one of the ladies has the doll up like this—" she holds an imaginary baby in front of her, "and she's looking at the baby and saying, 'I just love you so much. You are the best thing that ever happened to me!' And I thought, oh man, that's just so beautiful."

"So maybe you can try giving your mom a doll," Judy says to Dave. "Try bringing her a cuddly one."

"I don't know," Dave says, shaking his head, "Every time we visit her, it turns into, 'I want to go home,' and 'You're just like all the rest, all the liars!' She called my wife all kinds of names, and that's what got to me."

"Well, I was glad to see you let go of it today," Judy says.

"That's the first time," he says sheepishly, and wipes at his face.

"There will be many more," says Judy, "and this is the place to do it. You never have to be embarrassed about that."

19

SIGNS

DAVE SCHISSLER IS JUST UNDER SIXTY. His wife Kathy is a bit younger—too young to qualify on her own for the fifty-five-and-over community where they live. Dave and Kathy relax on the sofa of their Florida home. Gray-haired Dave wears jeans and a collarless tan shirt. Blond Kathy sports a pair of slimming black sweat pants and a black t-shirt with Curvalicious written across the chest. She laughs and explains that she works for *Curves*.

We are here to discuss Dave's mother, Thelma, who is ninety-two years old and living in Arbor Village. Thelma's move to Florida from Maryland is a recent development. Her move into the nursing home is also new, and according to Dave and Kathy, it was completely unexpected.

"She was in senior housing up in Maryland," Dave explains, "so she lived by herself—"

"She had her own little apartment," Kathy interjects.

"—until about a year ago," Dave continues, "and they kicked her out, because she started wandering the halls, rapping on doors and disturbing other residents."

Kathy says, "She kept telling people, 'The building's falling down. Get out!'"

I ask when Thelma was diagnosed with Alzheimer's.

Dave and Kathy look at each other and roll their eyes at the same time.

"She wasn't," he says.

"We didn't know," Kathy says, then she looks at Dave. "Was she officially diagnosed up there?" She doesn't give him a chance to answer before admitting, "We're not real clear, because his sister took care of her until nine months ago. We would only see Thelma periodically. Dave would talk to her on the phone every week, and he'd say, 'I don't know . . . she sounds like she's getting out there.'"

"She probably had it for quite some time," Dave admits. "But how would we know? I always thought when I talked to her on the phone that it was her hearing. I'd call her on Sundays and say, 'Hey Mom, how're you doing?' And she'd say, 'Who's this?'" He scrunches his nose and snaps out the words in a Wicked Witch of the West voice. "And I'd say, 'This is your son! It's me, Mom!' I kept telling her, 'You need to get a damn hearing aid!' I thought that's what the problem was. I thought that's why she was confused.

"I said to my sister, 'Why don't you get her a hearing aid?' and she said, 'Well, at her age it would be a waste of money.' I said, 'I think if she could hear, she could understand. Let's just get her one.'"

"His sister was in charge of everything," Kathy explains.

"I went to Radio Shack one time while I was up there, and I bought these little amplifiers, but she lost them in her apartment somewhere. I was never there long enough to take her to a doctor to get a hearing aid. That would have taken more than a week. It just seems like my sister could have done all that."

"They hardly talked," Kathy says, referring to Dave and his sister. "They'd been estranged for twenty-five years. That's why we didn't really know what was going on, because she had control of his mother's affairs."

"Yeah," Dave agrees. "We only talked after the apartment management kicked her out. Before then, my sister would do things like get my mom's groceries, but she wouldn't buy everything that was on the list. My mom always wanted mothballs, because she said there were bugs everywhere."

"There were no bugs," Kathy says.

"But she said the whole place was crawling with bugs."

"His sister must not have realized," Kathy says.

Dave admits that he had concerns. "One time I went to visit her, and we would have conversations, but they were confused. She would sit and talk with my Uncle Fred, whose picture was hanging next to her chair. She would have full-length conversations with this picture.

"That same visit, I was lying on the sofa in the living room watching TV. All of a sudden, her eyes started moving rapidly like something was going on, and she goes, 'Do you see them?' And I looked down where she was pointing and said, 'Do I see what, Mom?' 'That little boy and little girl sitting there at your feet,'" Dave says, imitating his mother's squawky voice as he points at the floor. "I said, 'I don't see nothing, Mom,' and she goes, 'They visit me once in a while.' And she was serious," he says, "like there was two kids there!

"The more I think about that visit," he admits, "I should have realized it was more than her hearing. If you'd open the refrigerator, there'd be a label on the milk that said, 'I know you're stealing my milk! Stay off!' or she had notes on the outside of the refrigerator that said, 'I know you've been in here! Get out!' She even had notes on boxes in the closet that said, 'I'll know you've taken this! I'll get you!'

"My sister knew about the notes," Dave confirms, "because she would bring in the groceries." He shrugs, then adds, "She must have thought my mom was just a worrywart or something."

"She had to have been in denial that this had been going on," Kathy says, "because when we got Thelma down here—"

"—it was kind of a shocker," Dave says, completing the sentence.

"She was really paranoid," Kathy says. "Ten years ago she started accusing her sister, Mildred, of stealing."

"They lived together for years," Dave says. "She would accuse my aunt of stealing her collection of birds, thimbles, money . . . everything was allegedly missing, from way, way back."

"And we believed her," Kathy says, "which is why we got her the apartment. We thought Mildred might have been going crazy and starting to steal from her. Now we feel kind of bad about that."

"She lived on her own in that apartment until as late as a year ago," Dave says. "She was convinced the building was collapsing, and that water was running down the wall. That's what she was telling people, which is why she got thrown out.

"The people who ran the place told my sister, 'If you don't control her, we will have to ask her to leave.' When it didn't stop, they gave her thirty days to move. My sister put her stuff in storage and took her home. They started looking into assisted living, but meanwhile my mother's wandering around my sister's house, and they were afraid she was going to fall down the steps.

"My sister's daughter didn't want her to be put in a home, so my niece thought, 'Well, I can take care of Grandma. I'll bring Grandma to my house.' She has three children."

"Little ones," Kathy says.

"So my mother went to live with my niece," Dave continues, "and my niece starts calling me up constantly—all different hours—crying and saying, 'She's crazy! I don't know what's wrong with her! She's up all night, and I can't control her. I don't know what to do!'"

Kathy jumps in, "It was all news to us that she was that crazy."

"After three weeks of pure hell, my niece had enough. She took her back to my sister's house and left her on the porch like it was a visit. She just slipped out and left. So now my sister is fighting to get my mother's clothes back from my niece."

"It was a weird situation," Kathy says.

"My sister is nine years older than me," says Dave, "and her husband is fifteen years older than her, so he's already an older guy. My sister can't take care of him and my mother, so when I heard how much they were struggling, I thought, 'I can do this. I'm going to go up and get her.'"

Dave insists that even after witnessing his mother's delusion and seeing the notes in her house, he thought she could live on her own.

"I started looking into assisted living down here. There was this guy at a place here who was really, really good in giving me advice. So I lined up a place for my mom and drove up to get her. This was just nine months ago. I didn't realize that I should have taken someone else along with me."

"The fiasco . . . ." Kathy says ominously, and they both laugh.

"We knew she was a little demented," Dave admits, "but nobody really recognized these signs all this time. We didn't know to what extent it was."

"We didn't know she had Alzheimer's!" Kathy insists.

"She knew she was going to come and live with us."

"And she was excited about coming," Kathy says.

"Right. So I got her in the car, and we took off. I'm thinking, 'This is going to be a good thing bringing her down her. I can do this. I'm doing the right thing.'

"I figured I'd drive eight hours, then spend the night somewhere along the way. I really had no idea to what extent it had progressed, because I hadn't been living with her. I just went up there and picked her up, and she seemed okay. I mean, we stopped and got donuts and had a coffee, and she was doing good. She seemed semi-confused, but sometimes we had moments of regular conversation.

"I said to her, 'You're really going to like it down there in Florida. The weather's so much better. You won't need a coat,' and she seemed to be pretty excited about it—until Florence, South Carolina . . . ." He slows down as he says the location, then slaps his palm against his forehead.

Kathy laughs. She knows what's coming.

"Once I pulled off in South Carolina, my mother goes, 'I know what you're doing. I know what you're going to do.'" Dave's voice is low and gravelly. "You're going to put me away!'"

"She just was out of it," he says. "When I was a kid, she never said cuss words—ever—but she got mean and angry and used words I never heard her use before.

"So we got to a Holiday Inn, and now she doesn't want to get out of the car. She said, 'I'm not going in there. I know what you want to do.' I don't know if she thought it was a nursing home, or what."

Kathy asks, "Had she started hitting you with the cane by then?"

"No," he says, "That was after."

Kathy laughs and lets him continue the story.

"It took me hours to get her out of the car. Hours. Then I went in to get the room. I kept an eye out the door the whole time. She was wandering around the parking lot, so I went out and I was pulling her, and she's screaming, 'He's robbing me! Robbing me!' and, 'He's raped me!' and 'He's a murderer!'"

Kathy says, "He's calling me on the phone, hysterical, saying, 'She's gone crazy!'"

"I had no idea. It was only later when I learned that people with Alzheimer's have this thing called 'sundowning,' where they get much worse around five o'clock. So, finally, I got her in the hotel, but she went up to the counter. They didn't know what kind of shape she was in, so when she said, 'Can you get me a cab so I can go home?' they're actually calling a cab.

"I said, 'Don't call a cab! She's got some kind of dementia!' They didn't know whether to buy it or not, but they didn't call the cab. She sat in a chair in the lobby and wouldn't move. People are coming in, and she's telling them, 'You have to be careful of him. He murders people. He stole my things.'

"I pulled two chairs together and just sat there looking at her to make sure she didn't do anything else. I could barely keep my eyes open."

Kathy says, "She went outside and flagged down the pizza man. She thought that was a cab."

"Later on, the night manager came in and offered to help get her upstairs. He said, 'I think she might have Alzheimer's. My grandmother had Alzheimer's.' So he recognized it.

"She didn't trust anybody, so I sat there 'til three or four in the morning. Finally, the manager convinced her to get in the elevator and into the room. She wouldn't let me lie down, though, because she kept smashing her cane on the walls and trying to break the window out with it. Then she'd swing it at me. She was more powerful than I would have ever guessed," he admits.

"I ripped the cane away and threw it under the bed. She was screaming and ran out in the hallway, no matter how I blocked the door with our suitcases. I know people had to be calling the front desk. So that went on for quite a while."

He and Kathy laugh.

"He kept calling me periodically," Kathy remembers. "I said to him, 'She needs a hospital. Call an ambulance.'"

Dave says, "But by that time I had called the guy from the assisted living place, and he told me there wouldn't be much they could do at a hospital. He said to just do the best I could—to do anything I could to be nice and calm her down. So I said to my mother, 'You want to go home? Let's go home.'

"Now the black lady who cleans the rooms comes down the hall. I went out and said, 'Could you just tell my mother that you need to clean the room and that she needs to leave?' She came inside, and my mother has this mean look on her face like she's been possessed." He bares his teeth.

"This girl is looking at my mother like, 'Are you all right? Do you want to leave?' And my mother goes, 'He beat me up! He hurt me!'

"She had a bruise on her arm here," he says, pointing to his upper right arm. "If you look at her arms now, she always has bruises on them."

"It's probably where he grabbed her arm when he was trying to get the cane away from her," Kathy says.

"So the housekeeper said to my mother, 'If you want me to call the police, I'll call the police,' and I'm like, 'Hold on a second here! What are you trying to do? This is my mother! She's got dementia or something!' And the lady's looking at me like, 'Who do I believe?'

"She gets on the walkie-talkie and calls for a manager. She says, 'We may need the police here.'

"By then, it was the day manager on duty, and he came up, but fortunately the police never came. This guy also knew someone who had Alzheimer's, and he was able to gain my mother's trust enough to get her to come downstairs. Everyone was real nice, and we got her in the car."

Dave looks at Kathy and they take a deep breath in perfect unison.

"So I'm in that car, and I'm out of there," Dave says with a wave of his hand. "She kept trying to unlock the doors and pull the window down. I had to hold my finger on the buttons so she wouldn't roll the window down." He pushes an imaginary button as he describes the scene.

"Now she's got that stupid cane again, and she's rapping me with the cane while I'm driving. Then once we got off the main road and we started heading through these little towns, she's taking things in and out of her purse and calling me all kind of names. I'm still trying to hold the button so she couldn't get the window down, but she got it down far enough that she could throw stuff out the window. Next thing I know, she threw this little tin with about four hundred dollars' worth of medication that I'd just picked up with my sister, and it goes bouncing down the road. I wouldn't have stopped to pick up one single pill. I just wanted to get to Florida.

"I'm still calling Kathy while we're driving and saying, 'My mother just threw her pills out. Go straight to the hospital! Let them know what's going on. Make sure somebody's waiting there. We can't take her to our house.'" He shakes his head. "There was no way the neighbors were going to see this crazy lady."

Kathy laughs and says, "Every time he would call me, I could hear her ranting and raving in the background, just hollering."

Dave imitates the raspy voice again: "'I hate you! I hate you for what you're doing! I'll get you for this! I hope you rot in hell!'"

Kathy puts a hand to her mouth to cover her smile.

"She was really out of control," he says.

Kathy looks at her husband. "She asked you, 'Where are we going?' and you said, 'You're going to the hospital.'"

"Yeah. I told her, 'Something's *wrong* with you!' I had no idea it was Alzheimer's."

"We thought maybe her medicine was messed up," Kathy says.

"Because we hadn't been taking care of her, we couldn't really get a clear answer of what pills she was taking," Dave explains. "She was still taking care of herself until she got kicked out. I don't know how she was able to do it."

"He would call me every few minutes, and I'd hear her in the background going 'Raghh, raghh, raghh.'" Kathy makes guttural animal noises in the back of her throat. "It was like a possessed voice."

"Yeah," Dave says. "It was like watching *The Exorcist*: 'I hate you! I'll kill you for this!' And it was nonstop. I'd never seen my mother act like that. So she's thrown out her pills, but she's still going through her pocketbook, taking things out and putting things back. She's out of control and agitated, and that's when she pulls out the knife."

He pauses for effect, and Kathy giggles.

Dave explains, "All this time I didn't realize that in her purse—wrapped in a napkin—she has a steak knife, and now she's really angry, and she's going, 'I'll kill you! I'll stab you with this knife!'"

Kathy tells Dave, "Your sister told me she used that knife to open her packages of Depends."

"Really?" he says. "Well, at this point she's lunging at me with the knife. I grabbed it," he says, and he mimics how he wrestled the knife away from her with a twist of his wrist.

"I got it out of her hand and threw it into the back. It was really a bad situation. I'm calling Kathy and telling her, 'We cannot bring her to our house to live. Something is way wrong. It's not normal.'"

"We had the bedroom all ready," Kathy says. "We really thought she was in good enough shape to live with us for about a month until we got her settled in assisted living. We were going to pay for it, and had that all worked out."

"I barely made it to the hospital," Dave recalls. "I near ran off the road. We could have been killed."

"You didn't even stop to go to the bathroom," she reminds him.

He laughs. "She wanted to stop and go to the bathroom. I didn't care if she peed in that seat. I was afraid if we stopped again and she got out of the car, it would be hours until I could get her back in, so we just kept going. I had to go, too, but I just held it in."

"So after about eight hours in the car, we arrive at the emergency room and Kathy opens the door."

"I had a nurse and a wheelchair," Kathy says.

"My mother was still angry."

"Yeah," Kathy says. "She was looking straight ahead, just as mean as could be. I opened the door and I said, 'Hi, Thelma.' and she said, 'Who are you?'" Now it is Kathy's turn to imitate the raspy voice. "I said, 'I'm Kathy,' and all of a sudden she was like "Oh! Ha, ha!'" Kathy goes limp and changes her expression to cheerful and smiling.

"She completely changed—just like that!" Dave exclaims.

"She was still kind of perturbed at him," Kathy remembers, "but she was very cooperative. If I hadn't heard her in all those phone calls, I would have thought he was the crazy one!"

"Fortunately she heard it."

Kathy laughs. "He had these little beady, red eyes from not sleeping. He was a nervous wreck. I never saw him look like that before."

"I was pretty messed up," he agrees. "I was exhausted. So Kathy took her inside the hospital, and she finally went to the bathroom."

"The emergency room ended up being an all night thing," Kathy says. "They got her admitted at like three in the morning. She ended up being in there five days until they could figure out where to take her next. About the third day, I'm sitting in her room and the neurologist came in. He was Indian, and he had an accent, so I thought he said he was a urologist."

Dave snorts.

Kathy flashes him an indignant look, then goes on. "People had told us that sometimes something as minor as a bladder infection can make people go off, mentally. So I'm thinking, oh, she must have had a bladder infection. We didn't know it was Alzheimer's.

"This doctor looked at me and said, 'She is very demented. How long has she been like this?' And I said, 'We just brought her to Florida. My husband's sister had been taking care of her. She had the Power of Attorney, but his mother has been living on her own.' And he said, 'You mean in assisted living.' And I said, 'No, she was in a senior apartment building.' He said, 'She wasn't in assisted living?' I said, 'No, we didn't understand that she was in this condition.'

"He said, 'It's not a matter of understanding, it's *acceptance!*' Kathy makes her voice deep as she mimics the doctor. "He was gritting his teeth, and he said, 'Why wouldn't you know that she was in this condition? This doesn't happen overnight. This has been going on for years!'"

She widens her eyes to show how stunned she felt by the doctor's words. "He said, 'This is a case of *neglect!*' And I said, 'We would go up and see her for Christmas, and my husband would talk to her every week on the phone. He said she was more confused as time progressed, but we just thought it was old age.'

"I told him that she took care of herself. Her place was clean, her laundry was done, and she was cooking . . . .'"

Dave jumps in, "Even though she had all these sticky notes that said, 'Get out of here! I know you're stealing!'"

Kathy shakes her head. "Her poor sister. Thelma said Mildred was stealing her money, and we believed her. She must have had a very slow progressing case, until now."

"She's progressing rapidly now," Dave says.

"So, Kathy was going around to find a place that would take her. Assisted living wasn't going to work. She needed to be in a nursing home. The people in the hospital almost jumped at me: 'You can't send a person like this to assisted living!'"

"We felt kind of bad," Kathy says. "It was hard for us to believe she had to go to a nursing home. She still made some sense when you talked to her."

"One nurse was really helpful," Dave says. "She came downstairs to meet with me. I told her we were having problems finding a home. We'd gone to a couple of places, and they said they had three or four beds. I'd go and talk to them, and they'd say, 'What's wrong with your mom?' When I told them she has Alzheimer's, all of a sudden they didn't have beds no more. It was almost like they were discriminating against her."

"We were denied because it was long-term," Kathy says.

"We're thinking, 'Suppose we can't find anywhere? What're we gonna do?' So this lady at the hospital said, 'I know a woman named Debbie Brazill. She's a really great person, and she runs a nursing home. Let me make a phone call and I'll let you know.' So they called me up just a short time later and said, 'We're going to be moving your mom today to a place called Arbor Village.'"

"I'd already checked it out," Kathy says.

Dave comments, "On first appearance, you'd think, 'This place is a dump!' but it's actually not that bad, compared to some other places that looked a bit more modern."

Kathy nods. "Like Dave, my initial impression was, 'Ooh, this is old,' but they take really good care of her at Arbor Village. They really care about the residents."

"Yeah," he agrees, "the people in there are pretty decent. They have some nurses in there that are absolutely amazing."

"His mom definitely belongs where she is."

Dave affirms, "The other day I was asking her questions to determine where she's at, mentally. I said, 'Mom, do you know your mother's name?' And she didn't. I asked if she knew her father's name, and she said, 'Frederick,' which was right, but they called him Fred. Then I said, 'Mom, do you know how old you are?' and she said, "I'm a hundred and forty-five, but they tell me I'm a hundred and ninety-nine.' I said, 'Mom, you're going to be ninety-three,' and she said, 'No, they told me a dollar ninety-nine!'"

"She wants out of there all the time. She says, 'Get me out of here!' She wonders how I got in. I say, 'I came in through the door,' and she says, 'You've gotta be careful. They're going to kill you. They're going to find you, and they're going to drown you in the lake!'"

"She's better when we go outside. We'll go to the fenced-in area to sit, and she says, 'We've got horses over there, and sometimes they're dead.'"

"She's talking about the goats," Kathy laughs.

"She thinks the goats are horses," Dave explains, "and she thinks they're dead if they're lying down. Sometimes she thinks they're dogs, sometimes horses. She just likes to go outside. She sits out there and talks to people walking by. It's quite funny, because there's a lady that goes around and around the sidewalks in her wheelchair. She stops by me when I'm having a conversation with my mother, and she says, 'Is this where you catch the bus to St. Louis?'" He raises his voice to a high-pitched squawk as he says the words. "I said, 'No you have to go around that way. You catch it over there.' And that goes on several times, over and over again.

"At the same time, there's a black lady who came over to me, and she goes, 'Have you seen my baby?' And I said, "No, I haven't seen any babies.' Then I kind of thought she was talking about those lifelike baby dolls. They've got like twenty of them, and they hold them and caress them. So I said, 'They're probably inside,' and she goes, 'No, they're not inside. They're out there.'" He points. "'Outside the fence,' she says, like she wants to get out. So, one wants to go to St. Louis and the other one wants to go out.

"Then you have this one other guy who wants to get out, too. There's three of them this whole time I'm visiting my mother. While one is trying to pull me out to go seek the baby, the other one is stopping constantly to catch the bus to St. Louis, and the other one is shaking the fence back and forth to try to get out. 'Is this where you get the bus to St. Louis?' he squawks again while Kathy laughs at his exaggerated antics.

"And this goes on and on to the point where it gets uncomfortable, because my mother's agreeing with all this stuff. She smiles, but there's no real conversation. Nothing makes sense, and it's a little freaky when they start pulling on you, because you never know what to expect. If you get them upset, how do you handle that? You don't know how to react."

"But nobody's been aggressive," Kathy says.

"No," he agrees. "I've never seen that, but the nurses say that may happen from time to time."

I ask Dave what spurred him to attend support group meetings.

"Some lady came up to me at the home and said, 'Oh, you just got your mom here. Are you new to Alzheimer's?' I said, 'Yeah,' and she said, 'Well, we offer a support group which I'm a member of. It's a great group, and you'll learn a lot if you come. You'll be surprised what you find out, because we all share information, and it may help you.'

"I didn't work on Mondays, so I figured I'd try it out. So I went one time and told the story about the trip down here, and they were all amazed. What surprised me was seeing the different types of people that were there. This one guy, Jim McBride, was married forever to this lady who passed away at Arbor Village, and he still comes to the meetings. Then you had the lady who was the director of activities there, and she ended up marrying him. So they both understand what everybody is going through, and they share their experiences.

"The things they would say sounded exactly like the things we're going through. I thought, 'Damn! That's what my mother does!'

"I'm still brand new at all this," Dave admits.

"I was real worried when I put my mother in the home, because I personally guaranteed the payment, not knowing how it was all going to work out, financially. So I go to one of the support group meetings, and they said they could hook me up with this person named Brenda Lee. I didn't know where to go or what to do."

"It was a paperwork nightmare," Kathy interjects.

"In that meeting there were two ladies who must have used her, and they're pulling the business card for Brenda Lee out of their pocketbooks." He points to imaginary people on each side. "So now I have information on where to start.

"This was really a good thing," he says, "because before that, we went to this attorney, and the first thing out of her mouth was,

'Well, it's going to cost you seventy-five hundred dollars for this, and it's going to cost you three thousand dollars for that, and what I would do is take all of your mother's money and go buy yourself a brand new car.' And I said, 'But I don't need a car!' and the lawyer said, 'It doesn't matter. You need to get rid of this money, and you need to do it now.'"

Dave twists his mouth. "So I said to her, 'But won't it look kind of weird if Medicaid sees that I've gotten rid of the money—like I'm hiding it?' and she goes, 'No, you tell them you're buying transportation for your mother.'

"I thought that was crappo information, and so I thought, seventy-five hundred bucks? She probably wants a big chunk of my mom's money, which wasn't that much anyway. So I called Brenda Lee from the home, and she actually came there that same day. She told me how much she charged, and it sounded good to me, because I didn't know where else to go. She gave me this list of documents she needed, and I brought them to the home the next day. I thought I was just going to be giving her the documents, but right there in that room she had one of her guys scan every piece of paper I had.

"She told me a lot of people didn't have half of the documentation I had available. I'd been making a binder so I could have everything in one place. They turned me over to another girl that worked for them. She told me what else I needed, and I faxed it to her. Just like that she said they had all the documents they needed, and that it should only take thirty days to get the Medicaid approved."

Kathy asks Dave, "Didn't someone tell you that your mother might be coming home with us after that initial hundred days was up?"

He nods. "I was real worried about that. I was thinking, what if I have to bring her home? What am I going to do? She'd been there almost the full hundred days, and the next thing I knew, they already had an approval. Everything fell into place."

"So that part was pretty easy," Kathy says, "but it hasn't all been that way."

She is talking about the mental aspects of adjusting to Thelma's condition.

"You see things that you're not ready for," Dave says. "Like when my mother comes out of the bathroom with nothing on."

"She would have never done that before," says Kathy. "She would have died."

Dave confirms, "She would never have done that. She was completely naked, and she had no clue I was standing there with her. I'm running out in the hall thinking, somebody's gotta help!"

I mention to Dave that he has been laughing as he has been sharing all of his stories, but that he broke down at the support group meeting.

"Oh yeah," he says. "I was in a bad way that day."

Kathy says, "He laughs to keep from crying."

It is not the first time a caregiver has said this.

Dave agrees with his wife. "You start off okay, and then you hear all these stories from other people like you, and it builds up. So when it's your turn, you break down.

"They ask me, 'What was your mother like when you were a child?' and I say, 'Well, definitely not like she is now.'" He shakes his head, serious now. "I mean, she's bad! She's totally different, just totally different.

"She has no moments anymore of being the mom I knew. That's not my mother in that nursing home. I've left there many nights and gone to my car and sat there and cried. It's unbelievable that she gets so angry at me and says things that no one would say to their own kid. She's angry and screaming at me, 'I hate you! I hope you rot in hell!' Then you have the nurses trying to control her and saying, 'Just go. Go ahead and just leave. We'll take care of her. Just leave.' And I go out and think, 'Who the hell was that?'

"So I get pretty upset," he admits, "but Kathy helps a lot."

Kathy gives him an appreciative smile, then says, "I would definitely advise people not to overlook it when they see changes in their loved ones. Look for things like paranoia, and if you just think they're getting a little forgetful, get more information. Pay attention to the signs."

Dave is back to laughing now as he shakes his head and says, "And when they start to talk to Uncle Fred on the wall, that's a big sign!"

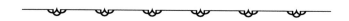

Judy turns to the last member of the support group who hasn't yet spoken. "Laura? How are you and Tom doing?"

Laura has a headful of curls and bright blue eyes. She moves that curly head as she speaks, letting those blue eyes meet each member present.

"Friends of ours came up who we haven't seen in a long time. They've known Tom from the very beginning of this journey. One of the men was there when Tom was first diagnosed, and he saw the stricken look on my face. Tom was kind of oblivious, and I said, 'We got a diagnosis of Alzheimer's.' This friend has problems of his own, and he took me aside later, and he said, 'Well, now you can be the angel to Tom that my wife has been to me all these years.'"

Laura's smile is peaceful. "That was so meaningful to me."

From the looks on the faces of those in the room, it is meaningful to them, as well.

20

BLESSED

I BUMP INTO CARMEN RICHARDSON at Arbor Village nursing home. She is there to visit her husband, Frank. We have already agreed to an interview, and she seems pleased now to have the opportunity to introduce me to Frank.

She leads me into a two-person room and greets a very large man seated in a wheelchair in the far corner. He looks to be at least six feet six inches tall with a good two hundred and forty pounds on his frame.

"Hello, dear," she says. "How are you?" She smiles as she bends down and kisses her husband. "I want you to meet a friend of mine." She turns to me, "Suzanne, this is Frank."

I greet him, saying, "How are you today?"

"Yes, fine, thank you," he replies.

I comment on his Panama Canal t-shirt.

"We took a cruise across the Panama Canal," Carmen says. "We both like to travel a lot."

Frank nods and says, "Yes." His eyes are vacant.

"She's writing a book about why we're here, so she'll be talking to us, okay?"

Again Frank nods. "Okay."

"Did you know it's raining outside today?" Carmen asks.

"It's raining," he replies.

"Okay, dear," she says cheerfully. "I'll be right back."

His head lolls to one side, but his voice is pleasant as he replies, "Okay. Yes."

Carmen and I step into the hallway and finalize the date and time of our interview. She returns to the room where, based on what I have just witnessed, I feel sure that she will continue chatting pleasantly in spite of the lopsided conversation. The energy that Carmen exudes is nothing but peaceful, and it speaks of her affection for Frank. If she is upset about having her husband in a home, she hides it well.

She greets me one week later at the door of a neat, upper-middle class home. The ambience is peaceful and quiet, just like its owner. Carmen's black hair is trimmed as short as a man's, but it suits her well. Her dark Latin eyes show the same warmth she displayed earlier at the nursing home. We settle into chairs on an enclosed lanai overlooking a small pond, and she begins to tell me about Frank.

"We've been married for eighteen years. Frank is seventy-two, and he was diagnosed with Alzheimer's five years ago."

Five years seems like a short time for him to already be placed in a nursing home.

Carmen explains, "The disease was progressing long before that. Fourteen years earlier—around the time we got married—he had been talking about having some forgetfulness. He was like the absent-minded professor. He saw a doctor and was tested, but all he told me was, 'Oh, I have some black spots in my brain.' He never said with what or why.

"We knew nothing about Alzheimer's, so if the doctor told him, he didn't tell me. He started taking Aricept right away, which should have been my first indicator. The medicine did work. It slowed the disease, in my opinion."

She describes a succession of jobs that Frank held during this time.

"He would go after something, then not pursue it. He would back away or get angry, saying, 'Ah, that's not worth it.' I don't know if that was his personality or the Alzheimer's. He was a brilliant guy, but he would lose his patience very quickly, so he was let go from one job.

"He used to play tennis, but I noticed that his interest in things slowly diminished as the Alzheimer's took hold. Then, when we were packing and preparing to move here, he was getting more and more confused and short-tempered. It was like I was walking on eggs all the time.

"He came down here before I did, because I had to wait to retire. He kept getting lost. He couldn't find his way, but in a new place that's understandable. About a week before I got here, he took delivery of the furniture, but he couldn't figure out where things went." She gives a small laugh and confides, "That might be a male thing, too.

"We have a love of travel and in those travels I noticed he would become much more disoriented and angry very fast."

She explains that some of their last trips together had their share of problems.

"We were on a river cruise in Germany. It was a Christmas cruise, and it was very nice, but cold. The porter was showing us around, and Frank was behind me because he was slower. There was a couple that went out the door, and I think that somehow in his mind he thought that I had left the ship and gone, so he followed the couple. I didn't notice that he had gone. I looked around and couldn't find him. He had followed them without any coat into the town. Somehow he found his way back to the ship, but he was furious at me that I had left him!

"That was before he was diagnosed. I knew there was something wrong, but I had no idea what was going on. I was really beside myself. I was drinking too much, because I was uncomfortable with what was going on with him and with me. I was thinking maybe it was my fault, and I was internalizing it.

"A couple of times he went back to Tucson, to his ex-wife. She was trying to get him to leave me and go back to her. We'd been married over ten years, so I knew something was terribly wrong. He would just say, 'I'm going to Tucson,' and go. I said, 'If you want a divorce, go ahead. I can't live this way.'

"I went off the deep end. I was drinking more and more. At one point he called, and I was drunk, and I cursed him up, down, and sideways, and he came back. So I said, 'We have to do something.' I knew that I was developing a problem and that he had a problem.

"I went to Alcoholics Anonymous. That's a wonderful program. They helped me a lot. Then I went to his family doctor and said, 'He's got to be tested. There's something wrong here.' This was five years ago, like I said."

Carmen is dry-eyed and matter-of-fact as she explains, "First we went to a neurologist who said he had Normal Pressure Hydrocephalus."

The name is a misnomer, as there is nothing "normal" about this neurological condition that can cause symptoms similar to Alzheimer's.

"His sister had NPH," Carmen says. "She had surgery for it, and she was fine. I wasn't happy with the diagnosis of NPH with Frank. I always want a second opinion, so I thought the Mayo Clinic would be the place to go. We scheduled an appointment there with a specialist in NPH. Frank was tested, and they interviewed both of us. The doctor said, 'He has enlarged ventricles, which is consistent with Normal Pressure Hydrocephalus, but his problem is, he has Alzheimer's.'

"Since then there's been another doctor who said, yes, it was NPH, and it could have been treated, but now it was too late. So, that's added to my guilt. The doctor at the Mayo Clinic says the other guy doesn't know what he's talking about." Carmen tilts her head and makes a "*Who are you going to believe*" face.

"One of the first things the doctor said to Frank was, 'You cannot drive.' Frank was furious at me. The doctor said, 'Don't be mad at her. I'm the one telling you,' but Frank blamed me for being there in the first place. He constantly criticized my driving. I couldn't do anything right. I preferred to have him drive, and to reverse the roles."

She says that impatience was an issue. "Well, even now," she reveals, "because I'm not the most patient person in the world, and to deal with a child—" She flicks her wrist. "It's important to portray somehow what this disease does. When you have a child, you see the child grow and develop skills quickly. It's a joy to see them learn to tie their shoes. Going to the potty is a big event. You listen to them say their prayers. All these little, ordinary things done step by step from an infant into an adult, and each event is a cause for celebration.

"This disease does the reverse. They're going backwards. It's step by step losing the ability to do those little, simple things that are now a cause for pain and suffering, as the adult loses the ability to do normal things." Her hand forms a fist, and her eyes fill with water. "Many tears have been shed over this," she confesses.

"For the last year before he went in the home, he had become so possessive that he didn't want me out of his sight. I wanted to go exercise, and he would get very upset. When traveling, he'd get upset at the dinner table. He would be very slow walking around, and if he lost sight of me, then he'd get furious at me. In airports he kept insisting he could pick up the luggage, and when I said, 'Okay, fine,' he couldn't find it. The luggage would go by and go by and go by. Then I insisted on getting it, and I'm five-foot-four as opposed to his six-foot-six. So he was becoming more difficult.

"I was beside myself, because I had to dress him and tie his shoes. I didn't have to feed him, but he was getting messy. He was at the point where he could not go to the bathroom. He was having accidents. When he did go, it was as though . . . ." She stands up and demonstrates turning around as if to sit on a toilet. "He couldn't sit down because he didn't trust there was something behind him to sit on."

She holds up a finger, as if she has just remembered something. "On another trip we were in Capri on a small, rocky boat. Part of his illness attacked his eyesight, and he was unstable. Getting off the boat, he missed the handhold, and he fell into the Mediterranean. They had four guys fishing him out. We had to laugh after we realized he wasn't hurt, but that was an indicator of his inability to interpret what he was seeing, and his gait got progressively worse.

"So he had fallen several times," she explains, "and he hurt his legs one of those times. He was in terrible pain. We went to the doctor, and he prescribed pain meds as well as therapy, but Frank wasn't getting any better. It was agony to see him drag himself from a chair. He didn't seem to grasp using a walker. Because of his size, he couldn't use a cane.

"A lot of times you'll hear there's a precipitating event for putting someone in a home, and he fell going to the bathroom. He knocked out the toilet paper holder and hurt himself. I called 9-1-1. They took him in, checked him out, and sent him home. Two nights later he fell again. They came, and they said, 'Do you want us to put him in bed?' I said, 'No, you've got to take him in.' I was pretty desperate.

"I'd been talking to a friend in the healthcare business who told me I had this window of opportunity for him to be placed. In the state of Florida, if a person is hospitalized for three days and the doctor sees there needs to be some rehabilitation, Medicare will pay for up to thirty days in a rehab facility. Then, after thirty days the person can stay and Medicare will pay eighty percent for a longer stay.

"I asked the doctor about it, and he said, 'Yes, we're keeping him for three days.'

"At the hospital, Frank was very belligerent, to the point where he had to be tranquilized. He was angry because he didn't quite understand why he was in the hospital, even though he was in a lot of pain. From there he went to the home. That's been a little over a year and a half.

"That's the hardest thing that anyone faces," she says, "to accept that they will never be coming home. Any change of environment is very disruptive to them. I hadn't realized that when we went traveling."

She gives a small jerk with her head. "Let me tell you about the last trip we took. We were going to go around the world." She laughs and rolls her eyes. "We had always talked about a world cruise, and I had to do all the planning. This was two years ago, and I was a little concerned about how the disease was progressing, but I thought it could work. I got all the visas and inoculations and did all the packing. The cruise started out of Los Angeles, but I didn't want to fly to LA with all the luggage for a hundred-and-twenty-seven-day cruise. So I said, 'Why don't we take a pre-cruise and minimize the disruption?'

"We got on the ship in Fort Lauderdale, and between there and LA I realized we could not continue. He fell three times. The ship, as big as it was, still rocked, and he couldn't get in and out of the bathtub. The last time he fell, the doctor said, 'You can continue, but we're going to go farther and farther away from medical attention.' He told me that ultimately the responsibility was mine."

Carmen admits that by then she had to dress Frank and do everything else for him.

"So we flew home from LA. The cruise line was wonderful. They shipped all the luggage."

She shakes her head. "Frank always said, 'They say I have Alzheimer's, but I'm fighting this. I'm okay. I'm okay.' Even now he says that, and that's a good thing—to not be aware. To be in a facility like that . . . ."

She sighs. "As nice as it is, it's still a holding facility. To realize they're going downhill . . . . I suppose if he were aware, he might have been able to help himself. He never realized how bad he was getting.

"I try to see him every other day. I stay about two hours. I feed him, I shave him, I brush his teeth. Sometimes he clenches his teeth and says no. That's one of the little acts of rebellion they have. They don't have many chances to act under their own control. I do his nails, I give him a neck massage, I read the newspaper to him, but that's pretty depressing, so I read *National Geographic*, which he likes. There's not much he can talk about. It's a monologue, and I'm not a big talker myself.

"On the one hand, I feel guilty when I leave there. Now, it's not so hard, because he seems to accept it. Before, I had to trick him and tell him I was going to a meeting and I'd be back. He doesn't seem to have the concept of time. I still say, 'I'll be back,' but not the same day. There's a sense of relief that I'm leaving a painful situation, because it's not just seeing him that's painful, it's all the others in there who know me—these lost souls . . . lost fragments of people."

None of these feelings showed on Carmen's face when we met at the home, but she reveals her thoughts now.

"To me, the real Alzheimer's is a condition that robs the person of who they are. It takes away their dreams. It takes away their personality and their memories. It takes away who they are.

"It's so important that people learn as much as they can about the disease," she says. "They should join support groups with others going through the same thing, because family and friends—as well-meaning as they may be—do not understand what the caregiver is going through. The patient, in my opinion, is living in a different world, and nobody really understands what that world is.

"I think that Frank is in a good place, in whatever world that is. He seems to be fairly content. Others that I've noticed—because I spend quite a bit of time at the facility—are in an angry place, a lost place, a place of misery and desperation . . . so each one is individual."

Carmen seems to catch herself sinking, and says, "There is some joy in all of this that Frank is still alive, so I would tell people to enjoy the good moments—those times within the limitations of the disease when you can smile. There are little things, like when I'm reading a story to him and I spur a comment from him where there's a moment of lucidity. Enjoy those moments. Enjoy the fact that they are with you."

She makes a short *tsk* sound. "It's a two-edged sword. I like those little moments, but on the other hand, I wish this were over, and he were gone, because he's not there. Of course, that makes me feel guilty . . . but not for long.

"It's important for the caregiver to accept that they have to go on with their life as best they can. I have a nice house, and my finances are pretty good, but I'm married," she tilts her head, "and I'm not married. That loneliness is there, even though I have good friends and I believe in Spirit. Thank God and the Universe that I've been blessed with the belief that there's more to this life," she says, looking upward, "and that I'm not alone. But even with that, there's a sense of being alone."

I ask if her spiritual beliefs have helped her through these difficulties.

She nods. "I believe that's why we're here—to gain mastery of ourselves . . . to learn these lessons." She gives a short sniff. "I should be a master by now, but I still have so much to learn.

"I consider myself blessed," she says. "Really, I'm blessed," and it is clear that she means this. "I'm blessed, because I'm learning about who I am. I am learning that I am larger than myself, and that there's a whole universe out there that's a very positive universe. I'm learning that I can deal with a lot and still feel blessed, and because I feel blessed, I seem to be able to do pretty well."

This explains the peace that Carmen exuded in the nursing home, in spite of the pain she has been describing here.

"People say, 'Oh, my goodness, you handle this so well! How do you do it?'"

She puts her hands out as if to say, "*It's obvious.*"

"We are one—you and I," she says, "and I feel connected with other people in the deepest sense. I sometimes waver and struggle with that, but somehow I feel very connected with people. I've been able to experience that connectedness, which makes me feel whole. So, I'm connected with Frank, and with the others in the nursing home, and it's a connection to a larger Being—a larger Universe. I'm connected to God through this.

"I go to the Alzheimer's support group pretty regularly. I occasionally do things with the people in the group. They meet on Sundays for a social thing. We visit, and we may go out to dinner afterwards. I exercise a lot. I take day trips with Triple A, and I take courses with the Adult Learning College. I go to AA meetings, because I like the people and the philosophy. I go to meditation class, and I read spiritual stuff.

"Do I have joy in my life?" she asks. "Yes. I'm grateful that I can find some joy within the situation that I'm in. I'm grateful that my life will continue, and maybe because I've gone through this experience—this vale of tears—that I'll be a stronger person and able to help other people.

"It's important that people realize that there is some hope. My husband always wanted to donate his body to research. It hasn't worked out that way, but he has been registered with the brain bank, which is a good thing for people to do. So, maybe their brain can help other people, and help with eradicating this disease. That gives me some hope—some hope that when my husband passes, that his brain will help to find a cure.

"In the meantime, you deal with it, but you go on with your life. Don't let it disable you. Don't let it be so consuming that it destroys your life now or afterwards. I wish it were different, but it isn't, so I accept it."

Carmen Richardson gazes at the peaceful pond beyond her window and says, "I'm going through this as best I can, with a feeling of gratitude that I *can* get through it, and with the awareness that there is something larger than myself. There's no question that I feel blessed. This has been a growth experience—very painful at times—and it's still ongoing. It's not a punishment, though, as some people would believe, but a part of my life's journey. So, I accept it as such, and know that it's an opportunity for me to grow."

———————————

Judy glances at the clock. It is time to end the meeting, but Laura is still talking. Judy remains silent, allowing her to finish.

"My friend said to me this visit, 'How are you coping? Your life is so different,' and I said, 'I think it's all in how we're looking at this. You can always find the weeds, but you can't always enjoy the flowers if you're always looking at the weeds.'"

Judy smiles like a teacher listening to her prize pupil.

"I firmly believe it's my relationship with God that's allowing me to deal with this," says Laura, "and sometimes—you all know—I deal with it a lot better than others."

Laura's fellow caregivers return her knowing look.

"It was a wonderful visit," she says, as the meeting comes to an end. "It really was."

21

LET YOUR LOVE SHOW

DOROTHY MCBRIDE OPENS THE FRONT DOOR. She is small in stature, but she exudes a large, welcoming glow far brighter than her colorful print top and white slacks. Her husband Jim towers behind her in the doorway, a gentle giant looking over his wife's head with quiet curiosity.

They welcome me into the cozy, neat house and lead me down a short hallway. Just as we get to the kitchen, Dorothy stops.

"Before we start, we want to show you our den. It's special." She glances up at Jim with an almost childlike sense of anticipation.

I follow her past the living room and turn left. Jim trails behind us, leaning on a brown cane for support. We enter a room with a wooden sign on the door that reads Dorothy's Buttery.

Dorothy explains, "I'm interested in pioneer days, and that's a term used by the lady of the house in those days. There was this room—the buttery—and it was very small. It had one chair and a small table, and the lady was surrounded by these shelves with all the canning equipment. It was her refuge."

She sweeps her arm through the air, introducing me to her buttery. "I've always had a room that was just mine. My husband had his den, and I had my buttery, but I have a fancy one now."

Dorothy's buttery has not one desk, but two; not one chair, but two. The walls are filled to capacity with photos, paintings, and memorabilia. She flashes a grin at her husband and says, "Jim calls it den."

He shrugs and grins back.

"We've been married a year and almost a month," Dorothy explains, so we blended two households. It's very important to us that our loved ones are part of our lives, and that's why we wanted to show you this room."

She leads me to the far right corner. "This is Jim's area, and this is his wife, Jean." Above a framed certificate and a drawing of the White House hangs a large, painted portrait. The woman in the picture has a full head of wavy, blond hair, as opposed to Dorothy's dark hair streaked with gray. She shows a round, pleasant face with a peaceful expression.

"And this is my area," Dorothy says, indicating the opposite corner. "And that's my husband, Bill."

A framed black and white photograph shows an equally pleasant man in a coat and tie. His head is balding, as opposed to Jim McBride's white hair combed straight back on top.

Dorothy points out several framed pieces of embroidery on the walls. "Jean did beautiful needlework. This one always hung in their guest room, and this one hung in Jim's office . . . how many years, hon?"

"Oh, about twenty years," he replies.

They lead me out of the room and back toward the kitchen. Along the way we stop again.

"And I do want to show you this beautiful picture," Dorothy says, pointing to a piece that occupies a central position in the living room. It shows a young girl sitting amid pots of flowers. The detail and shading are impressive.

Jim flips on a light so I can see better, and Dorothy says, "This is counted cross-stitch that Jean did. I do counted cross-stitch, but I've never seen stitches that fine."

We continue on to the kitchen and take a seat in three wooden chairs at a table pushed against a large window.

"Jim has a beautiful story," Dorothy says.

"I do?" he asks, looking pleased.

She smiles back at him sweetly, then tells me, "I'm seventy-six and Jim is eighty-six."

"Together, we have a hundred and seven years of experience," he says.

"We were both blessed," Dorothy nods. "We both had happy marriages: sixty-three years for Jim, and forty-four for me."

She explains that her first husband died unexpectedly of a heart attack at age seventy-two. "He's been dead now thirteen years. I had never imagined there would ever be another man in my life, but God had other plans."

They share a silent look. It is rare to see such open adoration between two people of any age.

"Jean was a patient at Arbor Village," Jim explains. "She was diagnosed with Alzheimer's about fourteen years ago."

"I was the Activity Director there," Dorothy says. "I met Jim, of course, because of Jean. He was just another family member at that point, but the one thing I admired in him was that he was so faithful. He came every day. The only time he missed was if he was sick, and even then, only if he had to be in the hospital."

"That didn't happen too often, thank goodness," Jim says.

"If he was at Arbor Village, he spent his time with his wife. A lot of people don't."

Dorothy explains that family members will often go to see a loved one, but they end up spending most of their time with other visitors.

Jim shrugs. "Being married sixty-three years, we had to stay together. It was always fulfilling to me to be there. I generally went in the morning and left when they took her to lunch. I'd go home and do whatever I had to do."

Suddenly, the rims of his eyes turn bright red as if being colored by an invisible paint brush. His eyes fill with tears, and he reaches for a tissue from a box by his elbow. "I'm a crier," he says with a hangdog smile as he removes his glasses and wipes at the tears.

I ask what led him to put Jean in the home.

His lower lip juts forward. "I just had to get some sleep every now and then. She wandered at night. She'd leave the house, and the neighbor up the street would bring her back. You had to keep an eye on her, otherwise you'd get out of bed and realize she wasn't there with you. So you'd get up and go and try to find her. That's when you'd thank the Lord that the neighbor brought her back. That happened half a dozen times, but we had a good life, and this is why I couldn't understand people having the problems they have."

"He's referring to the people in the support group," Dorothy explains. "We like to think we have a little wisdom to share, so we go every Monday, and that's what Jim's referring to—the problems that a lot of people are dealing with. He was blessed that he never had them, but every story is different."

"I never had problems with Jean," he says again, wiping more tears while Dorothy continues the story.

"It was part of my job to attend care plan meetings," she says. "That's when all the disciplines gather and they review the symptoms and how the patient is doing. I saw Mr. McBride at those meetings, and they were very hard on him. Those meetings just tore him up every month, so this one time I really felt sorry for him. I brought the tissues, and I said, 'Mr. McBride, you really don't need to come to these meetings if you don't want to. Make it easy on yourself,' and he agreed.

"To some people it's very hurtful when the nurse spells it all out, and that was what got him. We just became very good friends, and it grew."

Jim laughs. "Yeah, it grew. Being married for sixty-three years, I was pretty much set in my ways, but when I realized what Dorothy was . . ." he makes a devilish face, ". . . I thought, well, I'd better keep an eye on her. She's going to get in trouble."

She wrinkles her nose at him, then Jim grows more serious. "She was a friend, and not just a member of the support group. I felt like I could talk to her, but I never asked her out for a date or anything."

"No, because he was a married man," Dorothy says, as if stating the obvious.

"Her friendship meant a lot, but I didn't get to know her kids and she didn't know mine."

"But I knew his wife," Dorothy says, glowing with the memory. "When she first came to the home, she took a shine to me. She wanted to go home right at the beginning, then this one day she said to me, 'Do you live here?' and I said, 'Yes, I live here,' and she asked, 'Where?' and I said, "Right around the corner," which was where my office was, and that seemed to help her.

"The bond between Jim and me was special, too, because I knew the loneliness of losing my husband." Dorothy loses her composure for the first time, and her words are choked as she says, "I'd been a widow then about six or seven years. Jim had that same pain, even though Jean still lived.

"Any person that's dealing with Alzheimer's . . . it's a roller coaster thing," she says. "You go through happiness, and you hit the bottom more than once. It's the loss. They're in their body, but you can't talk with them. It's a very lonely road for the caregiver. Jim used to bring the Christmas cards that came in the mail, and they didn't mean anything to Jean, but he shared them with me, and that's how I got to know him and his family."

He has been listening quietly with the same gentle smile, his eyes never leaving Dorothy's face. Now, he joins in again. "I still had a wife and family, and it was always good for me to be there, but it hurt when I had to leave. That was daily," he says, tearing up again. "Oh yeah, it hurt every day. That's why I'm a weeper."

I ask if he was a weeper before his wife's illness, and he confirms this with a sheepish nod.

"But if Jean was having a bad day," Dorothy says, "he could always turn it around."

"See, Jean and I grew up together," he says. "We had known each other since the third grade. We were twenty-one when we got married, and it was a good life. We had two children—a son and a daughter."

"And I have two children," Dorothy says, "A son and a daughter."

"Jean was diagnosed seventeen years ago."

"Oh no, honey," Dorothy says. "Before that. I would think nineteen years."

He shakes his head. "No, I think seventeen was about it. We had gone on vacation to Indianapolis, and I had rented an apartment for a month. After we'd been up there one week, she got real antsy and couldn't sit still. Before we got there she was all in favor of staying for a month, but in the first week she'd had enough. She had to be doing something all the time, and it didn't make sense, so we just bundled up and came back home. I took her to a neurologist here, and that's when they came up with the diagnosis of Alzheimer's.

"I started doing the cooking, and I did the shopping and the laundry. She didn't have much of anything to do, and she didn't want to do anything, but there was never any problem. She never got out of hand." He wipes his nose with a tissue, wads it up, and drops it in a basket by his feet.

"She was always pleasant and even-tempered," Dorothy says. "She was a nurturer. She liked to nurture the other folks in the Alzheimer's unit."

"She was healthy right up to the end," Jim says, "and I was so surprised when they called and said she was gone. Apparently, she . . ." he searches unsuccessfully for the word. "I forget what they called it."

"Her body just started shutting down," Dorothy explains. "I always checked on her in the evening before I left, and I went to work this one morning, and they said, 'Dorothy, the hospice people are waiting for you.' They told me this was a rough one, because it was Jean, and she was actively dying.

"It was a big shock. Jean was very close to me, and they knew how close I was to Jim." She looks across the table at him, her eyes serious.

"All the deaths are rough, but this was more like my family. I loved her very much, and that's why it's important that we have those pictures in there," she says, glancing toward the buttery-den.

"I was privileged to know his wife. He never knew my husband, but they have made us who we are today. We share the same core values, and that was a reason not to be alone anymore. I've worked in nursing homes for thirty-five years, and nine times out of ten, when there's a diagnosis of Alzheimer's, the family members cut right away." She brushes her hands together as if cleaning them of dirt. "For someone to stay faithful like this is very unusual."

"For all those years there was nobody else," Jim says. "I wasn't out chasing around. I'd go home and go to bed and go right back out to We Care. That's what they used to call Arbor Village."

I ask how they finally got together. Dorothy glances down and laughs shyly.

"He asked me for my phone number, but I was reluctant to give it to him. I had his phone number, and I never called him, but I knew about being lonely after all those years. I finally decided that I would give him my number, and we talked a lot on the phone.

"Our first date was Christmas Eve. I invited him to my church for the candlelight service. That's my favorite service, and I wanted to share that with him. At first he said no, because his church was having a service at the same time, but on the afternoon of that day he called and asked if that invitation was still on."

She gives Jim a smile and says, "And that was the beginning."

He rolls his eyes. "And I've been in trouble ever since."

"We try to go to church at Arbor Village once a month. Jim went there every Sunday with Jean."

"For six years," he says.

"It was special for us," Dorothy says. "He would go to his own church after that. His daughter teased him that if he'd been better in his younger years, he wouldn't have to go to church twice in one day."

"Yeah," Jim says accusatorily, "You tried to manhandle me in that chapel." He turns to me and says with defiance, "I was in there, and she came and sat down beside me, and she almost sat on me— just throwing herself at me—and I couldn't escape."

They both laugh, and Dorothy shakes her head. "You're just *bad.*"

"We just feel like the good Lord put us together," Jim says, "but the one event that really brought us together happened back the day after Thanksgiving two years ago. I was living alone then, and I fell and wound up with both legs doubled under me. I couldn't get up, and I lay on the floor for over eight hours. Dorothy tried to call, and I couldn't get to the phone to answer it."

"That was one time my ESP came in handy," she says, "because I had the feeling that something was wrong. I always called him in the morning and evening, and when he didn't answer that one morning, I called back. I knew he could hear the answering machine all over the house, so I told him on the machine that I was on my way. Then I called my son. I told Kevin, 'There's something wrong with Jim, and I don't know what I'm going to find.'"

"They came over and found me lying on the floor," Jim says.

"He was fully clothed and he looked fine," Dorothy says, "but he'd been there all night. He was in very bad shape because he was dehydrated and his body was starting to shut down."

"They called 9-1-1. I went to the hospital and got all fixed up, but that's the reason I walk with a cane, because it messed my knees up."

I look at Dorothy and say, "You saved his life."

She smiles humbly.

"That brought us closer," Jim says.

"We were already dating then," Dorothy explains, "but that was the beginning of the beginning."

Jim nods thoughtfully. "It meant an awful lot to both of us that she could take care of me and get me the attention I needed." He pauses, looks into her eyes, then adds, "Now I'm stuck with her."

Their eyes sparkle as they laugh.

I ask Jim what kind of work he used to do.

"I was an electrical contractor, commercial and industrial."

"And Jean worked for a while," Dorothy adds.

"Yes, for Eli Lily pharmaceutical. I was one of those hard-headed Dutchmen that didn't think a wife ought to work, so I didn't want Jean working much and I didn't want Dorothy working after we married."

"I was seventy-five when I retired from my job at Arbor Village," Dorothy says with pride, "and I loved what I did. It wasn't work to me. From the first day I came home and told my family, 'I can't believe they're going to pay me to do this.' I just love working with the older people."

"It's a good thing," Jim says. "I'd be out in the cold."

Dorothy snorts and shakes her head. "I took care of my aunt Clara. She was the first person that had Alzheimer's in my family. To me, the real Alzheimer's is a person who has left their body. They're gone, and there's just this . . . ."

She pauses to find the right word, then sweeps her arm up and down as if in front of an invisible person. "They're just this body, but it's not them. There's nobody in that body. You can't talk to them, you can't do things with them. You can't share anything with them. That was in my family, and everything I was taught professionally doesn't help you at all when it's your own family. It's a different thing.

"Still, the nursing homes I worked in were not that huge, so you feel like each one is your family. It's an experience of pain and hurt all the time. It's very hard. If the caregiver has someone in a nursing home, they have no life. They go there, they spend the time, they go home, and usually they're exhausted. They lose contact with all their friends, and it's very hard to keep positive. Even though they put their loved one in the home, they're still not sleeping well. There's a lot of guilt to work through when you put someone in a home. I helped put Aunt Clara in." She shakes her head. "I can't imagine putting your spouse in.

"To me, it's the same thing as when you lose a spouse in death. You lose a lot of your friends. They don't know what to say or do, and they don't want to be around you, so you lose them. These people that I saw in the nursing home that I love very much, we encouraged them to have their own life, to try to build new friendships or repair some of the old ones . . . to somehow get involved.

"We have one in the home who has done this. She has a set of friends that we call 'normal,' and she has some that share the same path with the Alzheimer's, so she gets help from both. The important thing is not to lose yourself in this, and it's not easy. You have to always have hope. We never know when they're going to find a cure." She pauses, then points toward the ceiling. "Only the good Lord knows.

"Jim and Jean and both of their children had a very strong Christian faith," Dorothy says, "and I think that's what carried him through their troubles. His children were always supportive of any decision he made. He didn't have those problems like some of our friends who say, 'What are you doing putting Daddy in a nursing home?'"

"Yeah," Jim nods. "You'd be surprised how many friends you lose when you make a decision to do something, just like when Dorothy and I got married. I figured I lost some friends. They give you the attitude that 'Hey, she wasn't even cold yet, and you're out here with another woman.' It's tough to take, but you can read 'em like a book, the friends of yours."

"We still talk about Jean and Bill often," Dorothy says. "We keep our happy memories, and the only thing we've replaced is our loneliness. They haven't been replaced at all, because you can't do that."

Jim says, "To me, Alzheimer's meant a slowing down of our progress and of doing things together. We had always been very close, and we traveled a lot. The Alzheimer's put a stop to that, but we had a good life. I never had a problem with her.

"When I would go to the home to visit her, she would sit right there with me, but when it was time for me to go home, she'd take off down the corridor in that wheelchair like a bat out of hell and visit wherever she wanted to visit. I think she accepted the life that she had started to live. I couldn't complain, and this is what I can't . . . .'"

He stops talking to wipe at the tears that flow so easily. He drops the tissue in the basket, then shakes his head. "Working now with the support groups out at the home, I hear all these sad stories, and I didn't experience any of that. Sometimes I can't advise these people. All I can do is tell 'em, 'Hey, hang in there and love one another. Let your love show.'"

He reaches for yet another tissue.

Dorothy fills in the silence as he dabs at his eyes. "I think the hope is always that they're going to find a cure this afternoon, so you keep looking for these positive things. The human side of us never gives up. As long as they can keep on keeping on, it's part of their hope.

"The one thing I would say to other caregivers is that you are the healthy one. Live your life," she says, pointing her finger for emphasis. "And put yourself first. Eat first. Do everything first, before you care for your loved one. If you don't care for yourself, you're not going to be able to care for anybody.

"What would you tell them, Jim?" she asks, looking at him with undisguised affection.

"I'm bad at trying to advise anybody," he says. "I want them all to be happy, and to love somebody. That's the biggest thing." He chokes on these final words.

Dorothy comes to his rescue, saying, "He always tries to end our support group meetings with a joke. He says we've had enough seriousness; we have to laugh. And it's true."

She reaches across the table and squeezes her husband's hand. "There's no right way, there's no wrong way to do this. It's your way."

"That's right," Jim says, and his knuckles turn white as he squeezes back.

ABOUT THE AUTHOR

SUZANNE GIESEMANN IS AN AUTHOR AND INSPIRATIONAL SPEAKER. She is a former Navy Commander who served as a Commanding Officer and aide to the Chairman of the Joint Chiefs of Staff. With her books, workshops, and presentations, she now specializes in helping people bring more peace and happiness into their lives through love-centered living. For more information about Suzanne, visit www.LoveAtTheCenter.com.

Also visit: www.OneMindBooks.com

and: www.TheRealAlzheimers.com

ALSO BY SUZANNE GIESEMANN

Conquer Your Cravings

Living a Dream

It's Your Boat Too

The Priest and the Medium

Love Beyond Words

Messages of Hope

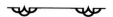

CO-AUTHORED WITH JANET NOHAVEC

Through the Darkness

Where Two Worlds Meet

The Real Alzheimer's

CPSIA information can be obtained at www.ICGtesting.com
Printed in the USA
BVOW081436071012

302232BV00002B/14/P